RESEARCH METHODS FOR NURSES AND THE CARING PROFESSIONS
Second edition

SOCIAL SCIENCES FOR NURSES AND THE CARING PROFESSIONS

Series Editor: Professor Pamela Abbott
University of Teesside, Middlesbrough, Cleveland, UK

Current and forthcoming titles

Psychology for Nurses and the Caring Professions
Sheila Payne and Jan Walker

Sociology for Nurses and the Caring Professions
Joan Chandler

Social Policy for Nurses and the Caring Professions
Louise Ackers and Pamela Abbott

Research Methods for Nurses and the Caring Professions (Second edition)
Pamela Abbott and Roger Sapsford

Research into Practice: A Reader for Nurses and the Caring Professions (Second edition)
Edited by Pamela Abbott and Roger Sapsford

Community Care for Nurses and the Caring Professions
Nigel Malin

Race and Ethnicity for Nurses and the Caring Professions
Ahmed Andrews and Lovemore Nayatangi

Nursing People in Psychiatric Systems
Chris Stevenson, Phil Barker and Shaun Parsons

RESEARCH METHODS FOR NURSES AND THE CARING PROFESSIONS
Second edition

Pamela Abbott and
Roger Sapsford

OPEN UNIVERSITY PRESS
Buckingham • Philadelphia

Open University Press
Celtic Court
22 Ballmoor
Buckingham
MK18 1XW

email: enquiries@openup.co.uk
world wide web: http://www.openup.co.uk

and
325 Chestnut Street
Philadelphia, PA 19106, USA

First Published 1998

A catalogue record of this book is available from the British Library

ISBN   0 335 19697 7 (pb)   0 335 19698 5 (hb)

Library of Congress Cataloging-in-Publication Data
Abbott, Pamela
     Research methods for nurses and the caring professions / Pamela Abbott and Roger Sapsford. — 2nd ed.
          p.   cm
     Rev. ed. of: Research methods for nurses and the caring professions / Roger Sapsford. 1st ed. 1992.
     Includes bibliographical references and index.
     ISBN 0-335-19698-5 (hb)   — ISBN 0-335-19697-7 (pb)
     1. Nursing—Research—Methodology.   2. Social Service—Research—Methodology.   3. Nursing—Research—Evaluation.   4. Social service—Research—Evaluation.   I. Sapsford, Roger.   II. Sapsford, Roger. Research methods for nurses and the caring professions.   III. Title.
RT81.5.S26 1998
610.73'07'2—dc21   97-42886
                                                                              CIP

Copy-edited and typeset by The Running Head Limited, London and Cambridge
Printed in Great Britain by Redwood Books, Trowbridge

CONTENTS

SERIES EDITOR'S PREFACE

It is now widely recognized that an understanding of research and research methodology is essential for caring professionals. However, while it is argued that nursing, for example, must become research-based, it is less certain that this is being achieved. Until caring professionals have an understanding of research methodology that enables them to evaluate research findings and utilize them in their own research, the aspiration for practice to be based on research will not be realized. Research-based practice relies on practitioners reading the research literature and implementing the findings in their own practice. It is now also necessary for them to be able to evaluate their own practice and the practice of others. Not all practitioners will become researchers – carrying out large-scale research is a specialized task that requires a high level of training. All, however, should be able to appreciate the research of others and understand how to incorporate research findings into their own professional practice.

This is a book on the appreciation and evaluation of other people's research and on the conduct of your own. It stands by itself but may also be read in conjunction with Pamela Abbott and Roger Sapsford (1997) *Research into Practice: A Reader for Nurses and the Caring Professions* (2nd edition), also published by Open University Press, which contains many of the examples which are discussed here. Both have been revised for this new edition; some of the examples have been changed, and the material on research into one's own professional practice has been strengthened.

One of the book's main aims is to 'de-mystify' research – to distinguish the often complex techniques from the basically fairly simple logic which underlies research projects. The focus is explicitly on social research: there is no attempt to cover research methods in biology, nor research into the efficacy of drugs. The principles are the same, however (except that social research tends to face more complex questions, because of the great variability of its subjects and the fact that the researcher is a part of the social world which he or she is investigating). Most of the examples are small-scale studies, in the sense that they could be (and in many cases were) carried out by one or two people rather than large and well resourced teams. Particular emphasis is given to evaluative research of various kinds and the attempt to assess the efficacy of one's own professional practice. (The term 'evaluative research' is preferred to 'action research' as defining the methodology for researching professional practice.)

Part of the target audience for this book is the nursing profession – people taking nursing degrees and diplomas, people taking post-qualificatory diplomas and certificates, and practising nurses who want to undertake research or the evaluation of their practice. For this reason a good proportion of the examples are based around the concepts of health and treatment. The book is also appropriate, however, for other community and institutional practitioners and trainees – for example, social workers, family workers, community workers. The intended level is introductory, and you should not imagine that reading it will fully equip you to carry out research of all kinds. (In particular, no attempt has been made to deal with getting funding for research.) There should be enough here to get you started, however, and the rest comes with practice, further reading and competent supervision by others who are already experienced.

Pamela Abbott

ACKNOWLEDGEMENTS

We should like to acknowledge our colleagues at the Open University, the University of Plymouth and the University of Derby, and elsewhere, with whom we have been teaching this material and discussing these issues over a long period of years. We are not aware of having 'borrowed' any of their ideas, but all academic work is an unacknowledged collaboration, and we have benefited greatly from having talked and worked with them. We can at least be sure, however, that the mistakes and unorthodoxies are mostly our own.

INTRODUCTION

FINDING OUT AND MAKING SENSE

Observation
Asking questions
Controlled trials
Research ethics and Research Ethics Committees
The research imagination
Summary
Further reading

'Research' is often presented as something mysterious and technical, something beyond the capability of those who have not undergone long training. It is what is done by scientists, it requires the use of computers and abstruse mathematics, and ordinary untrained people sometimes cannot even understand the questions, let alone the answers. However, 'doing research' is just an extension of what we all do in our daily lives. We are continually coming to conclusions on the basis of what we experience plus what we know already – to recognize something as a tree, or a post box or a person is to take knowledge which we have already and apply it to what appears to be in front of us. We all have occasion, every day, to try to find out more about something in order to act more appropriately – to look up an address, to take a closer look at the tree, to explore whether this person is really to be trusted. When something puzzles us and we cannot quite make it out, we generally set about looking for evidence about it which will help us to make sense of it. The researcher does no more. Research starts as an extension of common sense – finding out about things, looking for information about them, trying to make sense of them in the light of evidence and working out what evidence is needed.

Common sense has its limitations, however, which the researcher tries to overcome. In our everyday thinking and decision-making we often act on poor evidence. Indeed, we have to do so; events will not wait until the evidence is in, even if we were prepared to collect it. We come to quite hasty judgements about people, for instance, on the basis of one incident; we classify them as sympathetic or unsympathetic on the basis of how they behave when we first meet them, and behave accordingly. We judge whole classes of people on the basis of single examples. Common sense is full of 'facts' for which it has little or no evidence. What has been heard on the radio or television, or in the pub or the bus queue, or what is believed and announced by opinion leaders such as politicians, churchmen or scientists, becomes 'the truth' without further examination. Finally, common sense is influenced by a wide range of stereotypes and ideological presuppositions of which we are hardly ever aware. Our attitudes to the stranger, to the deviant minority, to those who might be seen as attacking our interests, are so well rooted as to be often impervious to the penetration of logic and evidence. The way we view the world is itself often open to question: our particular culture's construction of social class, gender and age as supposedly innate or inevitable stratifying principles – together with all the implicit assumptions about people and their wants and needs – are taken for granted as common sense.

Good research tries not to take for granted what is assumed by common sense. It tries to argue rigorously, according to the 'rules of evidence' which we shall be exploring in the rest of this book. At the same time, it requires a degree of imagination, and the power to put the taken-for-granted to one side and 'make the familiar strange'. It is not the *techniques* of research which make it hard work, as you will see in the rest of this book, but the strain of trying to see topic areas simultaneously from all possible angles.

The book falls into four sections. The first chapter is a 'mini-course', looking at most of the major ways of collecting data and structuring research and evaluation; it raises many of the issues to which you will come back again and again as you progress through the book. Chapters 2–7 are about reading and evaluating other people's research – Chapter 2 is about the structure of research reports in general; the others each take a type of research design and examine it through two or three major projects which have used it. Then Chapters 8–13 are on various aspects of the practice of research. The examples range more widely here, but some of them are drawn from the kinds of project that have been undertaken by students and could be carried out by you. Finally there is a chapter on the writing of research reports and a final summary chapter which also raises and pulls together more fundamental questions about ideology, discourse and the way in which the taken-for-granted aspects of everyday life are also taken for granted in research and evaluation studies.

We have provided practical exercises to back up the text wherever we can. If you are able to fit them into your lives, we strongly recommend trying to carry out the exercises, at the point at which they occur in the text; no amount of descriptive rhetoric is as illuminating as even a small-scale attempt at actually doing the research. The exercises are often quite short. Many of them either take no real time at all – they can be fitted into time spent travelling from one place to another, for example, or they can be accomplished in 10–20 minutes. Very few of them require any special arrangements or disturbance to your life, except when it is required that you ask someone direct questions, in which case you have to line up someone who is prepared to answer them – often a spouse or friend or working colleague. (The 'taken-for-granted' in the exercises is that you are able to leave the home in order to go to work or to the shops. If you are entirely housebound then you may need to modify some of them – e.g. observing family interaction rather than the interactions in shops or hospitals – but the exercises so modified will still make the points for which they were designed.) The exercises provided in Chapters 1 and 8–13 are practical activities. In Chapters 3–7 the exercises involve reading and commenting on particular research reports. These may mostly be obtained in academic libraries, or all of them may be found in Abbott and Sapsford (1997), the Reader mentioned in the Preface.

Various of the chapters also end with 'Further reading'. This is not necessary for the understanding of the text, but it is intended to expand your horizons beyond what we have written. In Chapters 3–7 the 'Further reading' suggests other articles or books you might like to examine if the subject area of one of the examples is particularly relevant to your interests or to your area of professional expertise – in other words, to research which you might be interested in carrying out. In Chapters 8–13 we mostly suggest further textbooks or articles which offer a more detailed treatment of the relevant research techniques than space permits here – plus a few studies worth reading because they use non-standard and imaginative ways of applying the method. These are not 'required' reading for the chapters, but additional material you will find useful if you go on to do research for yourself in the relevant area and/or style.

This chapter begins the book with a brief and cursory review of a wide variety of research activities, organized around the ideas of 'looking to see what is going on', 'asking questions' and 'trying something out'. We shall mostly be concerned here with questions of structure in research – structure in the way that questions are asked, or observations or measurements carried out, and structure in the sense of planned **comparison** between one group and another to illuminate their differences. (Throughout, words in bold are defined in the Glossary.) These are two dimensions along which research studies may differ. (A third major factor – how **typicality** or **representativeness** is guaranteed so that you can assert that what is true in the research context is true of the wider population – is left for consideration elsewhere in the book.)

Research is carried out for a wide variety of audiences. Much of what people think of as research – the kind of work carried out by 'researchers' – is to do with the evaluation of new or existing practices. Research is carried out to evaluate the outcome of a policy initiative or the functioning of an existing policy. For example, there will be a fair amount of research published in the next few years on how cash-limited budgets affect the practice of medicine, and on the functioning of hospitals before and after opting to become hospital trusts. In today's political climate of demand for 'value for money', research is undoubtedly also being carried out into the effectiveness of the health visitor policy of doing home visits to all homes with young children and on whether the expense is justified by what they do there. The effectiveness of treatments is evaluated by controlled research projects: the use of these is most obvious in the clinical trial of new drugs, but similar projects have also been run on the effectiveness of forms of psychological counselling, the introduction of new nursing practices and on innovations in social work practice. 'Before-and-after' projects are also carried out on social innovations (changes in forms of welfare benefits, for example) and gross demographic changes (such as the increased life-span of the population) on the 'clients' who are affected by them and the work of the professionals who try to help them.

A second major audience for research is the academic world. Much research is carried out not with the immediate aim of informing policy or practice, but to build an understanding of the field of study and to test theories about it which are derived from more general sociological, psycho-logical or economic models of how the social world is structured and how people function within it. Much of the classic work on health inequalities by region, class and gender, for example, may have been commissioned by government or more local authorities, but it has as its aim the discovery of factors associated with poor health, specifically whether the state of health of a group is more affected by their personal actions or by their position within society as defined by structural variables, such as class, gender and material deprivation. (This kind of research blurs into the more 'practical' work discussed in the last paragraph, of course; much social theory is directly concerned with the implementation of social policy.)

A third kind of work involves the evaluation of professional practice. (A fourth kind, less often thought of as 'research', but requiring all the same techniques, is the work of *self*-evaluation.) Research techniques can be used to evaluate the effectiveness of our own practice or that of others, and to test the effects of altering some aspect of it. They can be used to explore the wants and needs of client groups, so that practice can be better informed. They can be used in a vaguer but still rigorous way just 'to find out a bit more about' client groups and working environments, to see if any ideas are gen-erated which may be of use in our practice. This is something we all do without thinking of ourselves as 'carrying out research', but we can do it better if we apply a little rigour and logic. In many ways what distinguishes research from the common-sense use of argument and evidence is a certain 'cast of mind' – an openness to evidence and a distrust of presuppositions, even when taking this critical stance can be personally uncomfortable. When evaluating the work of others – whether their usual way of doing things or some innovative technique – we must clearly be seen to pass judgement fairly, without preconceived ideas, and on the basis of evidence.

In the rest of this chapter we shall be looking at some of the main ways in which evidence is gathered – **observation**, asking questions, and **con-trolled trials**. Practical exercises are provided for you to carry out, and you should try to find time for them if you possibly can; words on paper are no kind of substitute for actually doing some practical work and experiencing both the pleasures and difficulties of research. If possible, the practical activities should be carried out at the point in the chapter at which they occur, as the experience of doing them often acts to introduce or reinforce some teaching point which we want to make.

Observation

The most obvious way of getting to know a situation is to go and observe it, and observation is a major way by which research data are collected. Just how to do observation, however, is not quite as obvious as it might at first appear. Events are not just 'there' for us to note as if we were cameras taking pictures. On the contrary, in a sense we construct our world as we observe it, seeing what we do as a result of the knowledge which we already have. The same 'event' could be a parent disciplining a child in one frame of observation, a case of child abuse in another, and a piece of play-acting in a third. It could also be analysed in terms of local norms of parental discipline, patterns of communication or even patterns of physical movement. (One can – just about! – imagine a sports physiotherapist who was more interested in whether the muscles of the arm were working smoothly than in whether the hand was causing pain.) Similarly, there are many different ways of observing in research, ways which are good for different purposes and with different drawbacks.

Exercises 1–6: Observation

These exercises will take about 30 minutes, not including time spent taking notes. They do not have to be done all at once; they are split up into five-minute 'sessions', and each session could be done on a different day if that were more convenient for you.

Find yourself somewhere where the general public gather for some purpose and interact with someone who is in some kind of service or regulatory role. If you work in a hospital or general medical practice or in a social services department you may be able to observe a 'reception area' where people wait around for their appointments. If you are a health visitor you may be able to do your observation in a clinic. Parents may be able to observe other parents at 'mums and toddlers' groups. Otherwise, a good location is a large self-service shop where people take their own goods from shelves and queue at a cash desk to pay for them. Whatever the location, you want to find somewhere where you can stand around for five minutes at a time without drawing attention to yourself; those under observation must not know that you are observing, and if you are observing in a shop you will not want to be suspected as a potential shoplifter.

All the sessions require you to take notes. For the first two you will want to go away somewhere to do this – sit outside, or go and have a cup of coffee. The others require you to record numbers of various kinds, so you will need to take notes while actually doing the observation. Work out how to do this unobtrusively beforehand – in a small notebook, perhaps, or on what might be taken for a shopping list, or on a magazine or the margins of a book.

Exercise 1
Spend five minutes just looking round and seeing what is going on in general. At the end of the five minutes, go and sit down somewhere, and write some notes on what you have seen – not more than a page, but at least eight or ten lines, describing what was going on.

Exercise 2
Spend another five minutes focusing on the cashier or receptionist (without attracting his or her attention), looking at how he or she deals with people, how the people behave and whether they appear satisfied, disconcerted or annoyed by the interchange. Again, go somewhere and write some notes on what you have seen.

Exercise 3
Now spend another five minutes (or as long as it takes to get at least ten interchanges between the cashier/receptionist and a member of the public) looking at what is done in each interchange. Count how many of the interchanges involve one or both parties speaking, whether the cashier/receptionist appears to treat them in a friendly, distant or haughty manner, and whether the members of the public appear polite, rude, brusque or neutral to him/her.

Exercise 4
For another five minutes (or ten interchanges), count the total amount of time spent speaking in the interchanges by (a) the cashier/receptionist, (b) male members of the public and (c) female members of the public. Count slowly to yourself at a constant speed while any speech is occurring and jot down the numbers in three columns, to be totalled later.

Exercise 5
Spend five minutes concentrating on the cashier/receptionist, and count the number of seconds he or she spends looking at the face of the member of the public with whom he or she is interacting.

Exercise 6
Finally, go to another kind of location and repeat the count you have just done on a different cashier/receptionist. If you used a waiting room of some kind for your main location, go to a shop for this last part of the exercise. If you used a shop, try observing in a library or a garage or at the ticket office of a large railway station.

The notes from the first exercise, where you were recording simply 'what was going on', would probably tell us more about you than about the events which you were observing. What we asked you to do, effectively, was to make sense of the situation, and you will have done so largely in terms of your own well tried and pre-existing categories. It is possible that what actually happened may have surprised you, but nonetheless you will have described the situation in terms which came readily to you and made sense to you. You can see, however, that this kind of 'holistic' observation – trying to make sense of situations as a whole – is not as easy as it looks, and that more careful work needs to be done before the conclusions are readily acceptable as evidence. When we come to look at this kind of observation later in the book, you will see that it generally involves quite long periods of immersion in a situation, as a person with a role within it rather than just as a 'neutral' observer.

The second exercise may have taxed you more, because we asked you to concentrate on one participant for five minutes, a longer span of attention by far than you would normally grant to one person with whom you were not in interaction. This being so, we suspect you probably came to regard what was going on as to some extent strange – to start describing it to yourself in different terms from the ones that you would use in everyday life – and to that extent you may have come up with something which surprised you and would surprise us. Making the familiar strange is one stance regularly adopted by researchers who wish to penetrate below the taken-for-granted aspects of the situation. However, note that the closer focus on the cashier/receptionist in itself imposes structure on what you may have 'seen'; you were asked to focus on an individual, so you undoubtedly came up with notes bearing on the actions of that individual and the actions taken towards him or her, and with very little on the more general and structural features of the situation.

Exercises 3–6 introduced a new dimension by asking you to count something. What you counted became increasingly more specialized. What the numbers allow you to do is to provide a more convincing and 'available' description of the situation. We no longer have to rely on your judgement as to what was going on, however good and reliable that might be; you presented us with figures on some aspect of the situation, and we can look at them for ourselves. In Exercise 4, for example, we can see whether men spoke more than women, not just accept your judgement that one or the other gender was more active, and we can compare the activity of clients with the activity of the 'gatekeeper'. Comparing Exercises 5 and 6, we can look at the different behaviour of 'professionals' in two contrasting situations, as judged from an aspect of behaviour which has been shown to be very important in the regulation of face-to-face relationships.

Looking back over what you have collected, you will probably find that the data from the later exercises were much more 'definite' than what was collected in the earlier ones. ('Data' means 'what has been collected for analysis' – in the early exercises your notes on what happened, and in the later exercises the counts that you made.) Figures seem somehow to carry more weight in an argument than one's vaguer general impressions, to look more like 'proof', to seem somehow more 'neutral' than more general descriptions. You will realize already, however, that there is nothing magic about numbers as such. Numbers can, indeed, be more precise, and it is certainly easy to argue from them that something is more common than something else, or that two somethings are related. The value of the numbers, however, is created at the stage of data collection, and it depends entirely on your accuracy (how good were you at counting seconds?) and on what we decided to count in the first place. If what we decided to count was not important, then the data will be of no importance, irrespective of how neatly laid out in numbers they are. We constructed the situation as one in which speech and eye contact were 'the important thing that was going on'. All manner of interesting actions may have taken place during the interactions, but in the later exercises you will not know what they were. (At least, you may know what went on, but they do not appear in your data and are, therefore, not available for subsequent analysis.) Different frames of analysis – in terms of economic exchange, multi-person systems, personal histories, structural inequalities, etc. – are effectively ruled out by the way in which we elected to collect the data in the earlier exercises.

Thus there are many forms of observation, ranging from the very general and unstructured to the very structured and numerical. None of them is necessarily the 'right' way to proceed; each has advantages and disadvantages for particular situations, depending on your aims as a researcher and what you know already. We shall explore observation techniques in more detail in later chapters.

Asking questions

Another obvious and everyday way of proceeding, if you want to know what is going on and what people are thinking, is to ask them. A great deal of social science research is concerned with the asking of questions, and a substantial technology, folklore and body of expertise has grown up around the art and science of asking them. We ask a lot of questions as part of our everyday conversations. Ordinary everyday conversation can be a prime source of information, and you might well be taking advantage of it as part of a relatively unstructured piece of observation research. If you were studying a hospital ward without the people there knowing you were doing research – pretending to have an official role there, for example, or actually being a nurse and observing your own workplace – then part of the data you would collect would be what people said to you. If you were participating but being open about the fact that you were a researcher you could ask more questions, and more obvious ones; indeed, you would be expected to do so by the other participants. The strength of this kind of ordinary, everyday questioning is that you get what the participants want to say, in their own words and using their own concepts.

The problem with ordinary conversation is that you contribute as much to it as does the person to whom you are talking. Indeed, as it is you who are asking the questions, you will probably contribute more of the ideas that matter; it will be you that 'starts the ball rolling' with each topic, and the terms in which you do so are likely to structure the subsequent exchanges. So, far from getting the participant's own ideas in his or her words, you will get your own words and ideas fed back to you. An example which springs to mind is a student whom one of us was supervising on a methods course who was asking questions about social class and how the informant saw the social world as being structured. The informant used a categorization of working-class people into 'rough' and 'respectable', which the student found quite exciting, because it duplicated a set of categories which have been in use for over a hundred years and underlies the practice of charitable and state welfare – the distinction between the deserving and the undeserving poor. Checking back over the transcript of the interview, however, he found that he had been the first person to introduce this distinction, without thinking or noticing. The informant had found it a useful one and had used it consistently thereafter. So the student had no notion of how the informant would have described the world if this set of categories had not been made available.

When we 'interview' people rather than just chatting to them, we tend to play down our own part in the interview, to say as little as possible, to put across as few ideas new to the informant as possible and to concentrate on eliciting the pre-existent ideas of the informant in the informant's own words. This kind of interviewing is a very common means of research into social topics. It is often used to contrast groups of people who differ in some key respect or to compare the same people over time, and before and after major policy changes or 'social landmarks'. You will find it referred to in the literature as 'ethnographic', 'qualitative', 'semi-structured' or 'unstructured' interviewing. We did not like any of these terms, so we have coined the term 'open interviewing' to describe it.

So much for 'open' interviewing. There is also a more systematic and structured way of asking questions – you will probably be most familiar with it from being stopped by market-research interviewers in the street – which uses predesigned questionnaires or schedules. (A **questionnaire** is a list of questions for self-completion by the respondent; an **interview schedule** is a list of questions to be asked by an interviewer, face to face or on the telephone.) These are used in national **survey**s such as the Census for obtaining factual information from respondents – number of people in household, number of rooms in the house, etc. Their purpose is to collect exactly comparable information from every respondent, on a large scale. It is obviously important in the Census, for example, that the interviewers and respondents have a precise definition of what constitutes a household, and the same definition for every respondent. Otherwise, if the same group of people sharing a flat might be classified as one household in one part of the country and a number of co-resident single households in another, then we would be collecting information not about patterns of domestic living, but about whether people think of themselves as a household or not. Even an apparently simple question such as the number of rooms in house needs very precise definition. Does the bathroom count as a room? What about a separate and very small w.c., or a shower cubicle *en suite* to a bedroom? Is a breakfast room with a kitchen alcove to count as one room or two?

Structured questionnaires and interview schedules are also used for the collection of information about attitudes, beliefs and intentions, for example market-research interviews – 'What do you think of this product?' – and political opinion polls – 'Which political party would you vote for if there were a general election today?' Similar kinds of questionnaires are also used extensively by social psychologists and sociologists to test theories about the relationship of attitudes to each other, and they are one standard way of assessing likely popular reaction to policy changes. Their merit is that a great deal of data can be collected relatively quickly, and that the same questions are asked of everyone, allowing comparisons to be drawn. It is also possible, under certain conditions, to generalize with some degree of precision from a sample to the population as a whole; this is discussed in Chapters 6 and 9. There are corresponding disadvantages, however, as the following exercises may help to make clear.

Exercises 7 and 8: Interviewing

Exercise 7
Find someone who is prepared to sit down with you in a quiet place for a quarter of an hour or so – a friend or spouse will do – and ask him or her the following list of questions (for questions a–c, do not offer definitions

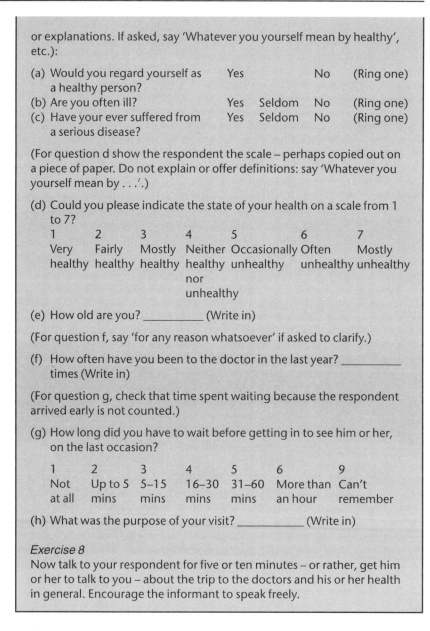

or explanations. If asked, say 'Whatever you yourself mean by healthy', etc.):

(a) Would you regard yourself as   Yes   No   (Ring one)
    a healthy person?
(b) Are you often ill?   Yes   Seldom   No   (Ring one)
(c) Have your ever suffered from   Yes   Seldom   No   (Ring one)
    a serious disease?

(For question d show the respondent the scale – perhaps copied out on a piece of paper. Do not explain or offer definitions: say 'Whatever you yourself mean by . . .'.)

(d) Could you please indicate the state of your health on a scale from 1 to 7?

1	2	3	4	5	6	7
Very healthy	Fairly healthy	Mostly healthy	Neither healthy nor unhealthy	Occasionally unhealthy	Often unhealthy	Mostly unhealthy

(e) How old are you? _____ (Write in)

(For question f, say 'for any reason whatsoever' if asked to clarify.)

(f) How often have you been to the doctor in the last year? _____ times (Write in)

(For question g, check that time spent waiting because the respondent arrived early is not counted.)

(g) How long did you have to wait before getting in to see him or her, on the last occasion?

1	2	3	4	5	6	9
Not at all	Up to 5 mins	5–15 mins	16–30 mins	31–60 mins	More than an hour	Can't remember

(h) What was the purpose of your visit? _____ (Write in)

Exercise 8
Now talk to your respondent for five or ten minutes – or rather, get him or her to talk to you – about the trip to the doctors and his or her health in general. Encourage the informant to speak freely.

The interview schedule you used in Exercise 7 is obviously a very short one, made up for the occasion, but it does display the major forms of question used. Questions a–c are essentially yes/no questions, though b and c offer a midpoint. (Did you have difficulty trying to get the respondent to say 'yes' or 'no' to question a?) Question d is an attitude scale. Questions e and f ask for a straightforward number. Question g again asks for a number, but the answer is recorded as a *code*, a number standing in for a range of possible answers. In question h you just write down (in summary form) whatever reason the respondent gives; this would be coded afterwards into categories.

The importance of clear instruction to ensure comparable responses is also evident. In most of the questions you were instructed not to offer definitions or explanations, but to force the respondent to make up his or her own mind what the questions meant. This would mean that the answers would have to be interpreted in terms of whether respondents think themselves healthy, not against some absolute standard of health. (We could have obtained further information which would have helped the interpretation of the data, however, by asking whether they had suffered from any of a list of diseases and ailments during the last year. Most people would describe themselves as healthy even if they have had a cold, for example, but only some would describe themselves as healthy, but suffering from arthritis.) We were careful to exclude 'unnecessary waiting time' in question g – time spent waiting because the respondent was early for an appointment. There are still ambiguities left in, however; for example, what about home visits from doctors, or times when the respondent visited the surgery, but saw the practice nurse, or visited only to deliver a specimen. At least one of the apparently simple counts is, in fact, fraught with potential error, because it asks for 'number of times in the last year'; people's memories are very unreliable for time periods such as this. (It might have been better to anchor the time period to a memorable event – 'how often since Christmas?', for example.) In that same question, you may have had difficulty coding the answer. What did you do, for example, with respondents who initially said 'not very long', or 'absolutely ages', or '15 to 20 minutes'? We didn't give you instructions on whether to probe or not – to ask follow-up questions. Did these responses go down as 'can't remember', or did you probe further to get a figure out of them? What confidence do you have in the figure, if they were vague initially? And note that if several interviewers were all using this schedule on different respondents, and they used different probes, then the answers to this question would not strictly be comparable. Designing structured questionnaires and schedules is not as easy as it may look at first sight.

When you talked with the informant afterwards, in Exercise 8, did you get the feeling that the definition of 'health' and 'healthy' was not the simple, cut-and-dried matter that the interview schedule seems to suggest? Did you, in fact, spend a certain amount of time *negotiating* with the informant what together you were prepared to count as 'being healthy', 'being unhealthy', 'being ill'? Did you find yourself swapping experiences with your informant and describing your own views on health? As you can see, the structured interview data are not nearly as rich and full as what can be collected by open interviewing, nor do they give one complete confidence that the respondent's complex views and life-circumstances are fully recorded. On the other hand, it would not be possible to use open interviewing on a very large sample: it takes too long. Also, you will have seen for yourself just how very difficult it is not to suggest to the informant what you are prepared to count as an acceptable answer – which would mean you were to some extent collecting your own views, not theirs.

Controlled trials

We have repeatedly talked about measurement before and after a change, and this is the key to the more systematic research design known as the **'controlled trial'** or **'experiment'**. If we want to try out a drug which is expected to reduce pulse rate, for example, it would not be much evidence of its effectiveness just to give people the drug and then measure their pulse rate; we could accidentally have picked people whose normal pulse rate was abnormally low or high. The minimum which would count as reasonable evidence of effectiveness, therefore, is measurements before administering the drug and afterwards, so that we could document a decrease. This is the essence of the experimental approach: a pre-test, a treatment or manipulation, and a post-test. Everything else that is built into experimental design represents the experimenter's attempts to show that the change is actually produced by what he or she says it is produced by – that there is no other plausible explanation for it.

In the simple drug experiment which we have just described, the evidence for a change is good, but the evidence that it is the drug which produced it is not very good. Almost anything might be responsible for it; for example, the group could have been taking exercise just before the administration of the drug, in which case we would have expected their pulse to decline from an initial high reading whether or not they took the drug. This kind of obvious physical feature can be controlled for – we simply make sure that it does not occur – but it is impossible to guard against every **confounded variable**, including those which have not even occurred to us. Normal practice, therefore, is to select a second group who go through exactly the same procedures as the first, but do not receive the drug. If pulse declines in the experimental group (the one that received the drug) and not in the **control group** (the one that did not), then we are on fairly firm ground in arguing that it is the drug that produced the effect.

However, this argument holds only to the extent that the two groups are exactly similar and undergo exactly the same procedures except for the experimental treatment. The experimenter goes to great length to ensure this similarity. Similarity of people is ensured by: **'matching'** cases (selecting pairs of people who are the same in key respects) and allocating one from each pair **randomly** to an experimental or control group; or by jumbling up the names of all the selected subjects, and drawing out an experimental and a control group at random; or sometimes by using the same subjects as control and experimental group. The merits of the three different approaches are discussed in Chapter 10. Similarity of treatment is guaranteed by careful duplication of procedures and by using a little imagination as to what might go wrong.

We have used a drug trial as an example of an experiment because such trials are easy to describe and understand. Precisely the same principles are applied in social experiments, however. Experimental social psychologists run just the same kind of procedure, with experimental and control groups measured beforehand on the variable which the experimenter intends to change, a 'treatment' applied to the experimental group but not the control group, and a post-test to assess the extent of the change produced in one group and not the other. You might use a similar procedure to assess the effects of an innovative nursing or social-work practice or the efficiency of a new teaching method. In the 'scientific' style of experiment, a key question is the accurate measurement of 'variables' – producing numbers which mean something, for subsequent analysis. The same design logic, however, would underlie an evaluation study carried out by one of the more **holistic** and less measurement-obsessed methods, such as unstructured observation or open interviewing. You would still want to assess how things were before the onset of whatever it was whose effects you were evaluating, and then again afterwards, and you might well include among the people you observed or interviewed a group who were not exposed to the change, to make changes among those who did experience it more interpretable by comparison.

Indeed, the same logic underlies many research reports which are not experimental. A frequent form of research involves looking at something which has occurred in one region – a new way of doing health visiting, say – and comparing some supposed outcome of it with how things were in the same region before the change and with how things were at the same points of time in a region where the change has not occurred. This cannot class as an experiment because there is no guarantee that the two groups which are being compared are like each other; regions may differ in the sort of people who live in them. You do have pre-tests and post-tests in both regions, however, and a 'treatment' administered in one region and not the other. The same form of argument would be used in interpreting the results, therefore, except that more care and investigation would have to go into demonstrating that it was fair to compare the two regions. (We sometimes call this kind of research **quasi-experimental**: it is *like* the experiment and shares its logic, but lacks some of its more important strengths.)

Exercise 9: Field experiment

At some time when you are likely to pass a fair number of people – on your way to work in the morning, for example – try controlling your own behaviour systematically and see if it has any effect on the behaviour of those whom you pass. With the first five people whom you pass, smile at them and look them in the eye. Note whether they smile back or greet you, and jot down the number unobtrusively – perhaps on the margin of a newspaper. (If you pass a group of people, focus on only one of them and do not count the others.) Now, with the next five, do not smile, and look at their chins instead of their eyes. Again, count how many smile at or greet you. Carry on doing this, smiling at five and not smiling at the next five, until you have at least 20 of each. Compare the number who smiled or greeted you in the 'smiling' condition with the number who did so in the 'not smiling' condition.

'Not smiling' is the control condition and 'smiling' the experimental treatment, in this exercise. As it was the same person who did both, we have no problems about comparing them in that respect. However, your journey to work is not uniform in terms of whether you are likely to meet people who already know you. Typically, people start off walking down a street where most people are known to them at least by sight, then get into territory less well frequented by acquaintances, then begin to recognize people again as they get near to where they work. This is why we asked you to do five 'smiles' and five 'no smiles', alternating: that way there is less likelihood that all of the people you pass in the 'smiling' condition would be known to you and all of the others unknown, or vice versa. Although only a small exercise, with a trivial 'manipulation', this design in fact shows many key features of the traditional field experiment of social psychology (i.e. one carried out 'in the real world', not in a laboratory or other artificial setting). It might have been set up to test a theory about the control of one person's behaviour by rewarding features of the others. On the other hand, it might have tested what happens when you initiate or do not initiate socially constructed 'greeting sequences' by catching someone's eye and smiling. Note that even where an experiment is technically well constructed, the interpretation of its results may not be unambiguous; in this case, the 'treatment' could be interpreted as two different things – administering a reward or initiating a 'social script' – depending on the theory from which you approach it.

You may also want to think whether the experiment was quite ethical. No particular harm was done to anyone, but it must have been disconcerting to some people to be, in a sense, greeted warmly by a complete stranger who then passed on down the street without following through into conversation. A charge often rightly levelled against those who carry out experimental research is that they are callous or unimaginative about the harm which their procedures might do to their subjects.

On the other hand, the overall logic of experimental design underlies all serious attempts to evaluate policy or practice. As we argued above, the *logic* of experimentation is not particularly tied to one method of data collection; it can be applied as readily to unstructured observation or open interviewing as to the more structured methods traditionally associated with it. Indeed, it also underlies a fair amount of conventional practice in the caring professions. The Nursing Process, or the Health Visiting Process, are modelled on evaluation studies and draw on their logic. They consist of a pre-test (assessment of a 'case' and his or her needs), a decision as to what is to be done, its implementation, and reassessment to determine the outcome. All that is lacking is a control group or condition. Social-work practice and teaching follow similar lines though in less explicit form; their practice consists of assessment of a situation, action in accordance with the assessment, and reassessment to evaluate the effects of action.

This process of evaluation, when used in research, has been referred to as '**action research**' by some commentators. However, we find this confusing and prefer the term 'evaluation research' – evaluating practice. Any of the research methods discussed in this book can be used to evaluate and inform practice. We prefer to restrict the term 'action research' to research structured so that its findings are continually fed back into the continuing practice situation and themselves become part of what is being evaluated. Again, any of the methods described in this book may be used. 'Action research', in this sense, is a sub-type of evaluation research.

Research ethics and Research Ethics Committees

In the previous section we asked you to consider whether the experiment we asked you to carry out was ethical. We are now going to consider the question of research ethics and the procedures for obtaining ethical approval in more detail, for virtually all research has potential ethical considerations – even when the research itself does not involve human subjects. This is especially the case for research findings, something over which the researcher has little or no control. Oppenheimer, after the United States dropped nuclear bombs on Hiroshima and Nagasaki, is reputed to have said that he would not have done research on splitting the atom if he had anticipated how the findings would be used. Similarly, social and health research can be used in ways which would be offensive to the researchers; for example, the results of research designed to find the most efficient and effective way of providing community care could be used by 'management' to justify reducing the nucleus of qualified district nursing staff and increasing the numbers of home care assistants. Researchers cannot always anticipate how the findings of their research will be taken up and used by others. The motives of a given research team may have been to improve patient care, but the findings might be used by management to impose new working practices and reduce staffing levels or modify the skills mix – something the researchers might believe would actually *harm* patients. It is important to consider how research findings might be used, but we would probably not do **applied research** at all if we refused to do research which could be used to justify actions other than those we intended.

What we are mainly concerned with here are the ethical considerations that need to be taken into account at the planning stage and the process of gaining ethical approval for research involving patients. All research that involves patients has to have Research Ethics Committee (REC) approval. Each district health authority has an REC, and approval has to be obtained for research from the committee(s) in whose district the research is being carried out. This may mean having to obtain 'ethical approval' from more than one committee. At an early stage in the planning of research it is a good idea to consult the secretary or chair of the committee and find out about the procedures for obtaining approval, which vary from committee to committee. Some universities also have ethical committees concerned with research on human subjects, and in some cases this committee or a sub-committee established for the purpose may have delegated authority from the health district's REC to approve the research proposals of staff and students.

The primary role of the REC is to review all proposals for research which involve any contact with patients or the medical records of present or past patients. The committee will be concerned about a number of ethical issues related to the proposed research. The University of Derby Research Ethics Committee, for example, has delegated authority at the time of writing from Southern Derbyshire Health Authority and uses the criteria in Table 1.1.

The Committee will also need to be assured that you have negotiated the

Table 1.1   Criteria used for ethical screening

How, if at all, will the health of subjects be affected?

Does the study have merit, is it feasible and practicable, thus ensuring that it does not waste subjects' time and effort?

Are there any possible hazards? If so, are facilities adequate to deal with them?

Is the investigation adequately supervised?

Are there acceptable procedures for obtaining consent from the subjects or, where necessary, their parents or guardians?

Will the subjects be given appropriate information on which to base their agreement to take part?

Are there adequate procedures for obtaining approval from the responsible consultant or general medical practitioner where appropriate?

Source: School of Health and Communities Studies, the University of Derby, School Ethics Screening Committee 1996.

necessary access with line managers before they give approval. In some health authorities there is also a Scientific Review Committee who screen proposals for the design and method of research and its likely contribution to knowledge.

Ethics are concerned with norms and values – standards of behaviour. They involve balance and judgement based on personal and professional knowledge and expertise. In research, ethics also relates to 'good practice'. There are no absolute ethical standards, but there are guidelines that can help us in deciding how to carry out research ethically and in evaluating the ethics of other people's research. Nurses have to adhere to the code of professional conduct of the UKCC (United Kingdom Council for Nursing, Midwifery and Health Visiting 1984). This states that

> Each registered nurse, midwife and health visitor shall act at all times in such a manner as to justify public trust and confidence, to uphold and enhance the good standing and reputation of the profession, to serve the interests of society and, above all, to safeguard the individual patient and client.
>
> (UKCC, quoted in Hammick 1996)

In addition the Royal College of Nursing issued a Code of Conduct for Nursing Research in 1977, the International Council of Nurses issued Guidelines for nursing research and development in 1985, and the Royal College added supplementary guidelines on confidentiality in 1987. A number of professional associations have guidelines for members: for example, the BSA (British Sociological Association), the BPS (British Psychological Society) and BERA (the British Educational Research Association). All of these documents can be useful in helping you to think about ethics and ethical principles when planning, carrying out and reporting on your research.

Hammick (1996) has devised a 'Research Ethics Wheel' divided into four quarters – practicalities of the research, the principles of the research, the duty of the researcher and the outcomes of the research. Issues to be considered under 'practicalities' include resourcing, the ability of the researcher to carry out the project, professional codes and the law. Those to be considered under 'principles' include the extent to which original knowledge will be obtained, respect for participants in the research and respect for authority. The issues relating to the duty of the researcher include veracity (truth), consent of participants, confidentiality and the weighing-up of risk versus benefit. In terms of outcomes, issues to be considered include the aims of the research, what happens to those who refuse to participate (or to those who form 'control groups'), the hazards and consequences, and the dissemination of findings. Hammick suggests that in reaching their decisions RECs pay most attention to issues surrounding informed consent and anonymity. These are key concerns because patients are vulnerable – they are unwell, often confused, and possibly compliant because the researcher or the promoter of the research is in a position of authority. It is essential, she argues, not only that informed consent is obtained but that those who are approached are informed in writing that non-participation in the research will in no way impair the care/treatment they receive, and that they can withdraw from participation at any stage. Patient Information Sheets written in lay language and readily understandable should be given to those who are asked to consider taking part. All those who agree to participate should complete a consent form. The REC would scrutinize the Patient Information Sheet and Consent Form before 'ethical approval' was given to the research. Another crucial issue is confidentiality/anonymity. Anything that a patient says when participating in research is confidential – it should not be passed on to others without the express consent of the patient. Similarly, research should always be written up in such a way that the anonymity of participants is preserved.

It is, however, necessary to recognize at the end of the day, as we said above, that ethics is about balance and judgement, and about justification. A key dilemma is whether the end can ever justify the means – for example, whether it is ever ethically justified to risk harming some people for the good of the majority. This has long been identified as a key issue in animal experimentation – whether it is justifiable to 'try out' cosmetics on rabbits to ensure that they are safe for humans. It also arises in medical research on humans, however – for example, in experiments where either a potentially beneficial treatment is withheld from one group or a potentially harmful treatment is administered to one group. In recent years the balance has tended towards ensuring that no human is harmed by research, but there can be no absolute guarantee of this, and if it were used as an ethical absolute it would prohibit all applied research. There are many other ethical dilemmas, and there are seldom 'right' or 'wrong' answers to them. However, whatever choices are taken, it is necessary that there be sound arguments in justification of them.

Exercise 10: Ethical questions

Consider the following questions and make notes on your responses. If possible, discuss your answers with colleagues.

1 Is it ever justifiable to withhold from participants the aims of the research?
2 Is it ever justifiable to carry out research when the subjects of the research cannot give informed consent?
3 Is it justifiable to use people as the objects of research?
4 Is it justifiable to carry out research that will solely or mainly benefit the researcher by, for example, leading to a PhD?
5 Is it justifiable to carry out research when the funders of the project retain the right to censor the findings?
6 Is it justifiable to accept funding for health research from the tobacco industry?
7 Is it justifiable to carry out research when the findings might be used to reduce staffing levels or to withdraw treatment from certain categories of patients?

Note: you need to give more than a 'yes' or 'no' answer to these questions. If you are inclined to say that a course of action *can* usually or often be justified, try to think of cases where it might *not* be justifiable. If you are inclined to think that it is *never* justifiable, try to think of valuable kinds of research which its prohibition would render impossible.

The research imagination

We have tended to talk on occasions, as everyone does, as if 'research' were a set of skills to be brought out and applied to the particular problem. This is true, of course, but a training in research entails more than this. As we suggested earlier, the 'research stance' is more a frame of mind, an openness and neutrality at the point of immediate argument, a kind of imagination. Few research projects are definitive in the answers they offer, and the unit of research is generally not the particular project – the **controlled trial**, the interview study, the period of observation – but the whole programme of related studies which explore and expand the question. Our notional drug trial, for example, would not be possible until the drug had been developed as a result of a large series of experimental studies in the pharmaceutical laboratory. Nor would one study be enough to show that it worked and had no harmful side-effects. The good research team would **replicate** – run the study again, to check that the results did not come up positive by chance alone. They would try the drug out on a wide range of people, to make sure it was safe for all and not just some of them. They would think about possible side-effects and run specific studies to try to detect them in a harmless form before they occurred in clinical practice with potentially fatal consequences. They would follow up all the people who had received the drug, over time, and look for longer-term effects. One question suggests another.

One aspect of the research imagination – particularly important in the more structured and 'quantified' styles of research – is having the imagination to know what data to collect. Open studies (participant observation, open interviewing) can often 'change their own agenda' by highlighting ideas as important which had not occurred to the researcher. More structured studies (questionnaire surveys, structured observation, controlled trials) solely collect the data they propose to collect, and are not open to surprises. To take an obvious example: if the classic **epidemiological** research on cancer had not collected information on whether people smoked, it *could not* have shown an association between smoking and lung cancer.

Studies may also lead to the research question being modified and expanded. In the case of the small field experiment you ran on the effect of smiling on the way to work, for example, we came up with two possible explanations – the 'reward characteristics' of smiling, and its function as the beginning of a well learned social script. If we were developing theory in this area we would want to run at least one further study to determine which of these, if either, was the more useful explanatory concept. In the process we might throw up further possible competing explanations which would need to be explored. We would also be developing our theory of the functions of smiling at the same time, and the developed theory might well suggest further questions which necessitated research. Where the questioning stops is an arbitrary decision; if the theory has merit, it is probably capable of indefinite expansion and refinement.

The researcher who does commissioned research also learns to widen the frame of reference when considering questions of research design. If you had been commissioned by management to study how cashiers in a large shop could improve the impression they gave to customers, or health receptionists the impression they gave to clients, you might well have carried out some or all of the observation studies which we tried out as Exercises 1–6. Management would have framed the questions in terms of what cashiers/receptionists do and how they behave, and social psychology's past research on the functions of eye contact and speech-sharing as satisfying aspects of interaction might well have led you to the kind of studies we proposed in the exercises. The underlying question, however, is not the narrow 'What can cashiers/receptionists do?', but the broader 'How can things be improved for customers/clients?', and you might well direct your research to this wider question rather than the narrower way in which management had framed it. The cashier/receptionist and her behaviour is only one element in the situation. You would have looked at her physical circumstances and whether they were conducive to friendly behaviour. You would have looked at the number of interchanges she had to manage – her workload – to see whether it was excessive. You would have looked at her rates of pay, and the rates of pay of comparable jobs, and the possibilities for promotion. You might even have regarded long queues as inevitable and looked at what was offered to clients/customers while they were waiting, to 'serve them up' as friendly people at the point of interaction. You would almost certainly have talked to everyone relevant to the

interaction – the cashier/receptionist, the customers/clients, other 'professionals' involved in the scene – to get their views and explore their satisfac-
tions and dissatisfactions.

The broader the frame of reference, within the practical constraints of
what can be managed within the available time, the broader the understanding, and broader understanding leads mostly to better solutions. It
takes a measure of imagination to conceptualize a problem widely enough
to make it really worth doing research on it. It is now some time since the
medical profession realized – occasionally – that more needs to be taken
into account in drug research than just the biochemical action of the drug.
(A famous series of experiments demonstrated that some doctors get better
results than others with the same drug, and that some doctors get better
results with placebos – inactive pills – than others get with the active drug.)
It is now commonplace in the teaching of nurses and health visitors to
stress that medical 'facts' about patients exist as just one part of complex
social lives and networks of understanding, and that what may seem a
good pattern of care from the medical point of view may not be the best
form of approach if the 'total patient' is taken into account.

Nonetheless, we lapse into simple thinking – not least in the sphere of
medicine and nursing – if we run simple studies based on preconceived
ideas of what 'must' be the right course of action.

The rest of this book is devoted to studying a range of good research
which has already been carried out, and to looking for ways in which 'good
practice' in research can be applied to the kinds of situations that you
might find yourself wanting to explore. We hope that you will bring your
widest imagination to the reading and not let anything be 'taken for
granted'.

Summary

1 'Doing research' is an extension of what we do in our daily lives –
observing, asking questions, trying things out, in order to make sense of
what is about us. Research starts as an extension of common sense.

2 Common sense has its limitations, however – particularly, it is full of
'facts' for which there is no evidence, and it takes for granted, embodies
and reproduces our cultural habits of assigning people and events to
categories and taking prescribed action on the basis of them.

3 The researcher tries to overcome these problems by arguing rigorously,
according to rules of evidence.

4 A more important difference between research and common sense is that
the 'research imagination' requires an openness to negative evidence
and a neutrality at the point of immediate argument, however committed the researcher may be to particular outcomes.

5 All social research has effects on human beings – by the way the research
is administered, by the selection of problems for research and/or by the
use made of the findings – and so all researchers face ethical problems.

Broad ethical principles are that the researcher should not misuse any power he or she might have, that subjects/participants should not be harmed or inconvenienced, that their interests should be taken into account, that their *informed* consent should be obtained, that their anonymity should be preserved and that every attempt should be made to see that the research findings are not used to their disadvantage. Nursing bodies and other professional associations have issued guidelines and codes of conduct which elaborate on these principles and offer more precise advice. All research involving NHS patients or their records is subject to scrutiny by Research Ethics Committees, and the same is true in many universities for research on human subjects. At the end of the day, however, there are no right or wrong answers, and the problems remain for the researcher to tackle.

Further reading

Hammick, Marilyn (1996) *Managing the Ethical Process in Research*. Salisbury: Quay Books.

ASSESSING RESEARCH

READING RESEARCH REPORTS

The structure of research reports
Assessing research reports
Ethical and political questions
Summary

In this section of the book we shall be considering a range of different kinds of research through reading and analysing a number of published research reports. The current chapter stands as an introduction to this work and looks at the structure of research reports and how best to go about reading them. Some of what we say may seem abstract and difficult on first reading, However, the research skills which we are trying to get across will become clear as you carry on with the rest of the section, read our evaluations of the papers and start to evaluate research reports for yourself.

When we look at particular research reports in Chapters 3–7, a starting point will be a checklist of the topics which we shall discuss briefly in this chapter and consider in more detail in the remainder of the book:

1 Does the design of the research lend itself to the arguments which are based on it – can the conclusions follow logically from what has been done?
2 Could there be other explanations of the results, alternative theorizations which might characterize what has been found in quite different ways?
3 Could the results be due to variables which are '**confounded**' in the design, accidentally confused with what we really want to measure? Or could they be an artefact of the research situation?
4 What is measured? Are the measuring instruments **valid** and **reliable**? Does the choice of 'quantities' to measure close off certain kinds of explanations and predispose us from the start to other kinds? (This is a series of questions, but they are all closely interrelated.)
5 To what population may the results be generalized?
6 Was anyone harmed, embarrassed or even inconvenienced by the research?
7 To what extent are people treated as objects by the research?
8 In whose interests is the research carried out?
9 Does the way in which the research is framed embody **ideological** presuppositions such that the outcome is 'written in' or 'predetermined' by the original conceptual analysis and design?

10 Are the results of any conceivable interest? Can I use them in my practice?

This is a checklist of the questions that can be asked of research reports. Not all of them are relevant to all reports. What we have tended to do in this section when discussing each paper is to concentrate on the questions that are most relevant for evaluating that type of research, not every question that could conceivably be raised. (It is also important to bear in mind that the questions we ask of a research report are, in part, determined by the purpose for which we are reading it.)

The structure of research reports

A formal research paper is expected to have a simple and readily comprehensible structure. Every paper outlines, in order: what the question or field of investigation is (and, probably, why it is interesting and/or what is already known about it); how the researcher or research team have gone about looking at it; what the results are; and what the results mean. Thus you can reasonably expect that a published paper aimed at an academic/ research/professional audience will consist of:

1 an *Introduction* which sets up the question or problem, explains why it is of interest to theory, policy and/or practice, and probably reviews the 'literature' (previously published reports, etc.) relevant to it;
2 a *Methods* section – how the problem or area is to be explored;
3 a *Results* section – what was found out;
4 a *Discussion* section – what the results mean, what they imply, and any major reasons for treating them with caution.

Books vary more in their precise organization, but you would expect a similar ordering of content (except that some of the Methods material is often relegated to an Appendix at the end of the work, to save 'ruining the narrative flow').

The form of this kind of report will be familiar to you from school science: it is the format of the school laboratory report ('Method: a pipette was taken . . .'). Not all 'social science' research would think of itself as 'scientific' in this sense, but the form of the scientific report is, nonetheless, a good one for presenting research results and showing what may be concluded from them, and it is widely used. This kind of report fits in most naturally with 'quantitative' research – **experiments, controlled trials, surveys,** systematic observation – but a similar *logic* is followed by reports of research in more 'qualitative' or 'appreciative' styles – open interviews, unstructured participant **observation.** What these latter tend to add is a greater narrative element, telling the story of the research process in more realistic detail.

Those who adopt a more 'qualitative' research design tend to be more aware of their data as the outcome of a process in which they themselves participated, and in which their own attempts to make sense of the situation and those of other participants will necessarily have had a great effect on what is produced. Thus qualitative reports tend to display greater **reflexivity**: they reflect more on the process of the research, on how the participants made sense of it, on their own preconceptions and on how detailed events may have shaped the nature of the data. In fact, you will now find an increasingly reflexive stance taken even in the more scientific style of report, as the proliferation of formal methods courses makes a generation of researchers more aware of the extent to which people make sense of their situation and how that can shape the nature of the data collected. Reflexivity is a quite essential component of the more qualitative research report, however; it is the major means by which we can assure ourselves of the quality of the evidence, given that we were not there when it was collected.

The majority of reports and accounts of research, of course, are not 'research reports'. Most are written for administrators who need to use the results, or for commercial companies, or presented to a relevant audience in one of the 'popular' professional publications (e.g. *Nursing Times, Social Work Today, The Health Visitor, The Magistrate*) or reported in the popular press or on radio or television for everyone's consumption. Many of the reports you come across in these ways will not cover all the sections that we outlined above. In particular, 'popular' reports tend to give little or no detail of how the evidence was collected; this is seen as tedious for the lay audience and therefore to be avoided. To the extent that such detail is not given, however, we should be very chary of giving more than a tentative and provisional acceptance to what is claimed to be the conclusions of the research. Popular reports tend to expect you to accept conclusions on the authority of the researcher; you are not given the resources to form your own judgement of their validity.

Assessing research reports

In reading a research report and assessing the worth of its conclusions,

1 your first steps will be to look at the Introduction, to see what the researchers were looking for and why it is supposed to be interesting;
2 secondly, you will look at the Discussion/Conclusions (and perhaps the end of the Results section) to see what the authors claim to have found and what they think it means;
3 with this established we can go on to look a little under the surface of the results and assess the quality of the evidence as well as the quality of the arguments based on it.

Looking at the arguments and the evidence, the first step is clearly to assess their overall validity: do the conclusions follow validly from the initial arguments, given the evidence that is presented? At the same time you need to look at the research part of the paper – the Methods and Results sections – and see if *they* constitute a valid argument. The paper will be arguing that certain kinds of results will be obtained or not be obtained, if an initial line of theory is to remain plausible. Or it will be claiming that an account of what a given social setting is like, based on survey methods or on open interviewing or on participant observation, is to be accepted as a valid characterization of what it is actually like. In either case there is an implicit argument in the project: 'given what I have measured or recorded, the best interpretation of it is the one which I am advancing'. You will be examining this claim very carefully to see whether alternative explanations could be put forward – alternative theories, or explanations based on inadequacies in the design of the research. Questions of reflexivity arise here; is the researcher well enough aware of the likely effect of the procedures on the data, and has he or she given us enough information to judge this? A part of the examination will also cover the question of measurement: are the measuring instruments or methods of recording and classifying observations valid – do they measure what the authors claim they measure? and are they reliable? are they likely to produce consistent results rather than values which are much at the mercy of chance? These are some of the questions we shall be exploring with you in the next five chapters, where we look in detail at a relatively small number of concrete research studies.

Another question which will arise in reading some papers – particularly the more 'scientific' ones – revolves around the question of **operationalization**. Many of the phenomena which the social scientist wants to measure are not readily and obviously available for measurement. What we actually have to measure is something which acts as a 'symptom' of the underlying characteristic – ability to answer questions on paper as an indicator of 'intelligence', job and/or attitudes (verbal expressions) as an indicator of 'social class', what patients say and what they do as indicators of 'depression'. From these we deduce a measurement for the underlying characteristic. The problem of validity which we mentioned in the last paragraph obviously applies: in translating the theoretical characteristic into something operational that can be measured, do we succeed in producing something which really does measure it? A further problem arises, however. Psychologists take the concept of intelligence for granted, for example, as we all tend to do nowadays, but the idea that people can be placed on a continuum of general ability in this way is a fairly recent invention (see Rose 1985) and one which embodies as 'fact' a range of politically very contentious ideas and practices (see Kamin 1974). Sociologists take their ability to place people in social classes for granted, and measures of social class are a commonplace in very down-to-earth projects such as the analysis by **market researchers** of what newspapers different kinds of people read. The way the concept is used, however, often presents as facts some very contentious statements about social inequalities (see Abbott and Sapsford 1987a, for example, for a discussion of the problems and consequences of assigning social class in different ways to married women). So, part of the assessment of a piece of research may involve **critical analysis** of its basic concepts – the apparently unproblematic 'things' which it sets out to measure – to see whether ideological presuppositions are being put forward unwittingly as unproblematic 'facts', biasing the outcome of the research from the outset. This kind of critical analysis is an aspect of the 'research imagination' about which we talked at the end of Chapter 1.

The other 'methods' question you would ask of any piece of research is to what population its conclusions are meant to generalize – of what is it supposed to be an example? Very little published research, even on single cases, is meant to tell us about just that single person or setting. (In this respect it differs from the case reports of the clinician or the social enquiry reports of the probation officer; these may be informed by the principles of research and, indeed, constitute a form of research, but they are seldom of sufficiently general interest to be worth wider publication.) Where a single case is researched, it is often chosen as being **typical** of some class of cases or at least as casting light on some class of cases; for example, an ethnographic study of one school will aim to tell us something about schools in general, or at least schools of that type. (Alternatively, the single case may be deliberately extreme and chosen to test a theory – 'if it is happening *anywhere*, then it is happening here'. The 'Affluent worker' study in Luton in the 1960s (Goldthorpe *et al.* 1969) was research of this type, selecting Luton as somewhere *un*typical of traditional working-class communities.

Most research extends beyond the single case to the sample – large or small according to the type of design – which is to be taken as **representative** of a designated population of cases. However, to take an obvious example, if all your research subjects are men then you would be unwise to generalize about 'the human race'; women might be different. Quite a lot of research has based conclusions about a culture or even about people in general on research into White males – either students or volunteers – and neglected questions of gender, race, age, class/wealth, geographical location, degree of physical or mental impairment, and all the other characteristics which might have made a difference to the results if only they had been considered. In assessing a piece of research we often have to be aware of quite subtle ways in which a sample might appear typical of a given population; it can in fact be unrepresentative because of the way in which it has been selected. So, another aspect of the 'research imagination' is that, if we are satisfied that the conclusions hold up for the case or sample under consideration, we still have to think about the extent to which they also hold up for the wider population of which the case or sample is said to be representative or typical.

Having assessed whether the methods and arguments of the paper are valid, you will want to return, with more confidence, to the paper's contents. Research is ultimately about substance – about the problems and questions which it explores – and not about its methods. Taking into account any reservations you may have as a result of your analysis of methods, what you will want to know is whether the paper tells you anything new and interesting. Does it add to or elucidate theory? Does it inform or criticize the operation of policy? Does it suggest anything which you can use to improve or modify your own professional practice?

Ethical and political questions

Finally, a further set of questions will also need to be considered as we build up an assessment of a piece of published research – Questions 6–9 on the checklist at the beginning of the chapter. Whether anyone was harmed or inconvenienced by the research is the basic 'minimum question' of research ethics: did the researchers act responsibly, leaving the world no worse a place by pursuing their investigation? We may reasonably go on to ask whether there is any benefit to the 'subjects' or 'informants' of the research, and whether the research is justified if there is none. This means, for example, asking in whose interests the research was carried out. Is it obviously commissioned by management, for example, to look into how workers can best be exploited – or dominated by that perspective, even if not formally commissioned? Is it to do with the social control of working-class people, or youths, or women? Is it set up to explore how the convenience of doctors or nurses or hospitals can best be served? More fundamentally, we may ask whether the research paid proper attention to the fact that it was *people* who were involved in it. Some feminists (see, for example, Reinharz 1979) have likened conventional social research to the act of rape: researchers go into a situation, take out of it what they need for their own ends (publication, academic esteem, promotion) and leave the subjects/respondents/informants at best not much harmed; they certainly obtain no benefit from the process but are there merely to satisfy the needs of the researcher.

These three questions do not affect the results – though they may affect our opinion of the researcher – but they lead quite naturally into a yet more fundamental one: does the way in which the research is framed embody ideological presuppositions such that the outcome is written in or predetermined by the original conceptual analysis and design? In other words, is there a very bad failure of the 'research imagination' in this research?

Summary

1 A very common way of structuring research reports is into the sections of the traditional 'scientific practical' report – Introduction, Methods, Results, Discussion. Research in qualitative traditions may depart from this ordering, but the same kinds of information will have to be delivered.

2 A logical way of approaching research reports is to look at: the Introduction to see what question is being posed and what the aims of the research are; the Discussion/Conclusions to see what answer is being given and the extent to which the aims have been achieved; and then at the Methods and Results to examine the evidence which sustains these conclusions.

3 Important 'methods' questions which will be asked of any research reports are whether the conclusions follow logically, whether the measurement procedures are valid, to what population the results can validly be generalized.

4 We would also want to ask ourselves whether anyone was harmed or embarrassed by the research, and in whose interests it was carried out.

READING OPEN INTERVIEW RESEARCH

The research paper: Abbott and Sapsford (1987b) 'Leaving it to Mum' (on
   mothering children with learning difficulties)
Discussion
Summary: points for evaluation
Further reading

> **Exercise 11**
>
> This chapter is based around Section 2 of Abbot and Sapsford (1987b)
> *Community Care for Mentally Handicapped Children* – ' "Leaving it to
> Mum": motherhood and mental handicap'. If you can get hold of this,
> you might like to read through it quickly before proceeding. A slightly
> shortened version is reproduced in the Reader which is designed to
> accompany this volume – Abbott and Sapsford (1997) *Research into
> Practice: A Reader for Nurses and the Caring Professions.*
>   While reading, bear in mind the list of questions suggested at the
> beginning of Chapter 2; it will also form the basis of our comments
> below. (However, we shall not try to answer every one of the ten
> questions for every one of the research papers on which we comment.)
> Also, make a list of the questions that you would have liked to ask us, if
> you had the opportunity, about how we did the research.

The research paper: Abbott and Sapsford (1987b)

This paper describes an interview study which we carried out in a new town
in the middle 1980s, plus some data drawn from Abbott's earlier doctoral
work (Abbott 1982). It is part of a longer monograph which also sets mental
handicap in its historical context and traces the development of government policy towards people with learning difficulties. (These were most
commonly called 'mentally handicapped people' at the time when it was
written; terminology changes as sensitivity develops and as situations are
re-theorized.) As you would expect, the paper starts with a brief exposition
of the 'problem' and why it is interesting:

The policy of 'community care' for mentally handicapped children has non-financial costs for families: work which in institutions would be wage-labour becomes unpaid work for 'Mum' when the burden of care is transferred to the family. This paper looks at the nature and extent of such work and at the extent to which it alters the nature of the mother's life. We look also at the price which is paid by the whole family for the fact of having a mentally handicapped child . . . (The 'price' differs markedly from family to family, depending at least in part on the degree of handicap, the extent of associated physical handicaps and the social and economic situation of the family: what follows is a composite, not necessarily true to the experience of any one mother.)

(Abbott and Sapsford 1987b: 45–6)

We are reminded, right from the start, that even though this is detailed 'open' interviewing of a very small number of 'cases', nonetheless what is to be presented is an average or typification, with some idea of the range of variability around that average, and not straightforward life histories of particular mothers.

The method of the joint interview study is described thus:

Sixteen families were contacted from a list extracted for us from the school rolls of two Special Schools in the new city (one designated for the mildly handicapped and one for the severely). We carried out two interviews with each mother separated by about a year, not using a formal questionnaire but rather trying for the atmosphere of a friendly chat about life and work between neighbours. Although the interviews were tape-recorded, it seems to us that this atmosphere was readily attained in most cases . . . These data are contrasted with a parallel series of interviews with mothers of children who have not been labelled mentally handicapped.

(p. 46)

So we know that the method was 'open interviewing' cast in a 'life-history' mould – asking women to describe their current and past lives, but steering them towards topics of particular interest to the researchers. We note that the 'sample' is not statistically **representative** – one would not wish to say that because half or a quarter of the sample said or felt something, then half or a quarter of the corresponding population were likely to do so. However, it is a reasonably **typical** sample in the sense that it shows a reasonable range of cases, in terms both of the ages of the children and of the degree and type of their condition, so any major problems (or any conspicuous lack of them) would probably be represented somewhere in it.

The account was written for a particular publication format, and its length had to be kept down, so many of the details which might have appeared have been omitted. The paper does not mention some of the strengths of the procedure. For example, we failed to record in the paper that we went in with an 'agenda' of basic questions which we wanted to cover somewhere in the interview. Though the questions were seldom or never asked explicitly, they served to make sure that key topics were covered by everyone, and that we did not form conclusions on the fact that someone had failed to talk about something important to us, when the fact of the matter was simply that it had failed to come up in the conversation. Chief among the strengths was the sheer **naturalism** of the situation. The interviewers were very evidently a couple, having 'got together' not all that long ago, and some of the atmosphere of a 'family visit' was sometimes achieved; it is remarkably natural for one couple to be talking to another mother about children and the experience of bringing them up. Pamela's pregnancy helped here. By the time Pamela had been settled comfortably in a chair and cushions arranged to support her, and Roger had been taken to one side and asked how she liked her coffee (a curious variant on the 'Does she take sugar?' phenomenon), some degree of acquaintance seemed already to have grown up. Later in the interview series some of the same effect was unwittingly achieved by the small child we brought with us in a carrycot, owing to the lack of babysitting facilities.

Among what is not recorded is some of the detail of the informants, the interviewing and how it progressed – this might have helped the reader judge its **validity**. The paper does not record, for instance, that the tape recorder did not work for the first interview, so that we were reduced to sitting down afterwards and writing out, independently, everything we could remember that was said. It does not record the number of tapes which were difficult to decipher afterwards because of the noise of children playing in the room or building work going on outside. It does not talk about the interviews which were difficult to 'get going', nor give much detail about the roles in which informants tended to cast us and how these changed. We do not talk much about the individual mothers, in fact, and this detracts from the richness of the presentation.

One of the findings we report, as you might expect, is that the mothers to whom we talked are very aware of their children's status as 'handicapped' and very aware of other people's reactions to it. Apart from the obvious reactions of strangers, even more difficult to deal with are the 'ignorant' reactions of friends and neighbours:

> When I talk to people and I say 'Mark is mentally handicapped', and as soon as they know he is coming up to sixteen, you see, you know what I mean? . . . You see it before they even say it . . . It is an unspoken look . . . there is that fear of danger to 'my daughter'.
>
> (Abbott and Sapsford 1997: 62)

Such reactions can be looked for even from within the family:

> Let's put it this way, there were relations we have not seen since we found out about Trevor . . . [and] we have only been invited to tea with Trevor once to my brother-in-law. He thinks we should put Trevor away.
>
> (Abbott and Sapsford 1997: 61)

The mother's life comes very much to centre round the 'handicapped' child, in a majority of cases. The amount of sheer physical labour – washing and cleaning – is immense, with children who will normally not become 'house trained' till substantially after other children – in their teens or never, in the most severe cases. Another part of the burden is constant supervision; as one mother pointed out, you expect to have to be home to supervise a 5-year-old, but not a 15-year-old. In many different ways these mothers' children caused extra work and took up extra time, and the fact that the labour was freely and lovingly given did not diminish its extent. In all this it was clear that the concept of 'community care' basically meant 'care by mother'. Some had help from neighbours, some from immediate household, some from wider family, but in many cases the help was intermittent or trivial, and in many cases it did not occur. Eight of the 16 families had no help from neighbours, and six of these also received little or no help from kin.

We also attempted a tentative typology of 'coping strategies' – trying to find a characterization of women's (or families') lives as a whole which would differentiate some families from others (in terms of the general style of their self-placement with regard to the outside world) and some women from others (in terms of the constructs they used to characterize and justify their lives). We noted a difference between those families which seemed determined that life should go on 'as normal' and those which conceded that there was something with which to 'cope'. Within the latter class we noted the 'bare copers' – those who managed from day to day and year to year – and those who seemed to have formed some stable kind of 'adaptation' to their situation. Within the latter class again we noted that some women seemed to have adopted the 'wife and/or mother' designation – seen as a positive role, not a form of constraint – as a preferred characterization of their current lives and as a description of their life goals. That is, they found themselves satisfied with what they were doing and appeared not to desire for any form of change.

We went on in this study – unusually for research into 'social problem' categories – to attempt a comparison with the 'normal':

> Shortly after the second interviews . . . one of us conducted a series of interviews with a 'sample' of mothers whose children had not been labelled as mentally handicapped, roughly **matched** for size of family and area of residence (which **correlates** well, in the new city, both with social class and with availability of 'social resource'). The sample is of course too small and haphazard to be representative of mothers in general . . . but the two samples match closely enough for some tentative conclusions to be drawn. One can after all say little about what is distinctive in the experience of mothering mentally handicapped children except by comparison with the general experience of mothering.
>
> (Abbott and Sapsford 1987b: 65)

Overall we found similar kinds of work being done by the two samples, with a similar lack of help from both community and kin, but the work was greater in extent and more demanding for the mothers of children with learning difficulties, and they received even less help from kin and community.

The biggest difference between the two samples of families came in the kind of future that they could foresee. In the normal course of events children grow up and leave home, and women receive back their power to dispose of their daily time. Children with learning difficulties do not necessarily leave home unless the parents actively determine that they shall do so, and the feelings of guilt and apprehension which are associated with the child's teenage years colour the whole view of the future. For some families the decision will effectively be taken for them by events: one or two of the children were so severely physically handicapped that they were not expected to live into their twenties. For others it was clear that a decision would have to be taken, in the child's interests. Some families were adamant that their child would stay with them, for ever if need be: 'When you think what her mental age is, say four or five, by the time she's nineteen she won't be more than that. You wouldn't stick a five year old in a hostel, would you?' (p. 74).

For many, however, the decision is a mixture of the child's interests, the convenience of the family and a feeling that in some way the problems of an adult 'child' are beyond what the neighbourhood can cope with.

Finally, the paper summarizes the study's conclusions about

> the real cost of bearing and bringing up a mentally handicapped child in the community. Some of it – the day to day grind of 'child work' – falls largely on the child's mother . . . The rearing of a mentally handicapped baby does not differ in kind from the rearing of any other baby – itself a substantial social burden – but it differs in its density and its duration . . . The burden goes on, moreover, potentially for ever, unless the decision is made to send the child away . . . Specific to mental handicap . . . are the other range of major problems which families encounter: the reactions . . . among strangers and also within the family and kin group.
>
> (Abbott and Sapsford 1987b: 74–5)

Discussion

In what purports to be an evaluation of research methods we have spent a fair amount of time looking at the substantive findings of the study – what it has to say about mothering children with learning difficulties. We have also given you additional information which was not in the report but which might be thought vital if the research is to be properly evaluated. This will not, of course, be possible when we are discussing the research of others. We cannot generally, when reading a report, ask researchers questions which might provide additional information about their methods and methodologies. It is therefore important, when writing up research, to consider what material about the methods has to be included to answer possible questions. Limitations of space often cause problems, however, and researchers often respond to them by leaving out the information which is vital for an informed evaluation of the research.

We read research studies mostly to look at what they have found out, not to study their methods. The study of methods comes in, however, when we need to determine whether we believe what is stated, whether it accords with the evidence as given, and whether the conclusions are possible ones given the ways in which the data have been collected. We need to look then to the strengths of each method, in general and in the particular case under examination, and to the corresponding weaknesses of logic of that type of research in general or this particular example of it.

One very definite strength of 'open' approaches to research – just talking to people, or observing and participating in their lives (discussed in the next chapter), without imposing much structure on what is collected – is the immediacy, the vivacity, the feeling of actually 'being there'. The Abbott and Sapsford (1987b) piece carries the actual words of the informants and lets them tell their own stories, often better than we could tell them for them. No amount of second-hand description can convey what it may be like to have a mentally handicapped child nearly as powerfully as the words of Mrs Miller:

> For about a month after I found out I didn't have any feeling for her any way – she wasn't my baby, she was just a baby that had got to be looked after and fed and kept clean . . . [And then] I walked past the pram one day and she looked up at me and she smiled at me . . . she just smiled . . . After that I was all right.
>
> (p. 47)

The price that is paid for this power and immediacy, which comes from the detailed study of a few cases or a single setting, is a necessary doubt about the representative nature of the 'sample'. To what extent does an interview study of less than 20 mothers of mentally handicapped children in one geographical location tell us anything about the problems nationwide of this kind of community care? In our study we did our best to 'cover the range' – to include as wide a range of 'cases' and social settings as was possible. We sampled, for instance, mothers from both a 'severe' school and a 'mild' school, so we could reasonably expect to contact cases ranging from near-total physical and mental inability to children who could have passed for 'just a bit stupid' at ordinary schools (and we did, in fact, contact cases covering this entire range). Our sample was well scattered through a new city in which geographical locality is fairly well correlated with social class and material circumstances, and we had everything from a mother permanently on social security to one in a substantial rural house set in its own grounds. Some of the sample were 'immigrants' of recent date to the new town, some had moved there in the 1940s and 1950s from London, and some were locally born and still to a large part involved in the original local 'village' community. However, we do not know how representative the new city is of places where parents whose children have learning difficulties might be living. Thus even if we are fairly confident that the results generalize to all families with a child with learning difficulties in that city, we would probably be less confident that they would generalize to families living in other parts of the country. Also, we do not know the extent to which looking after a child with learning difficulties is typical of caring for other groups of dependants.

We would certainly not want to assert that a particular percentage of all such mothers held this or that belief, or experienced this or that problem, on the basis of our handful of cases, but the problems experienced by our informants are probably not far different from those experienced by all such mothers. Nonetheless, all were 'customers' of the same schools and health and social service provision, so a study carried out elsewhere might well come up with different experiences depending on how much service differs across the country. Our study was also tied to a particular historical time, since when there have been major changes: we do not know how the newer policy of integrating mentally handicapped children into the 'normal' schools has affected the lives of mothers.

The other question which must be asked of this kind of research, where so much depends on the building of relationships and so much is apparently 'left in the hands of the informants', is the extent to which the findings are specific to those particular relationships, or even 'created' by something that the researchers did or said. The only guard against this, and the only warrant of validity, is constant **reflexivity** in the research and in the report of it – constant attention paid to what is going on, and detailed discussion of all aspects of the social situation and the procedures in the report. Our report is weak in this respect; it is characteristic of short reports of 'open' research that what is omitted in order to keep length down is the reflexive account, important as it is, and while reflexive material has been supplied, there is not as much of it here as we would have liked.

One aspect of reflexivity which you should look for in research reports is an awareness of the crucial importance of role and audience in the construction of interview data. 'What is expected' differs according to setting: the accounts we give when we are 'doing a public performance' are different from those we might produce in the privacy of the home. Similarly, a male interviewer may be faced with a different kind of account from what would be produced for a female, and the same goes for young *v.* old, Black *v.* White, able-bodied *v.* disabled . . . The account which we produce is very much conditioned by who we see the interviewer as being and, therefore, what is to be seen as 'relevant' or 'useful'.

Informants *have* to make sense of the situation before they can function within it, and how they do so is much conditioned by our presentation of the situation. They have to use the clues we provide to work out what we are after and what we see as relevant. One common way of introducing this kind of research task, for instance, is to present it as one which a student has to do as a requirement of the degree. The risk here is that to present the interviews as just a student task may devalue the work and lead the informants to produce accounts which are easy, memorable and picturesque, but not necessarily 'true' in any usual sense. The major alternative tack is to present the work as 'research', as in the Abbott and Sapsford (1987b) study, but the problem here is that the term 'research' is ambiguous in common language and has no single clear meaning. Our informants were quite clear as to why they were being interviewed: they knew they had been approached because their children had learning difficulties. Most started off by identifying us with some branch of the support services – as doctors, psychologists, social workers – and assumed that we were in some way checking up on the efficiency of provision. When they realized that these identifications did not hold up, we tended to become (in their view) the other kind of researcher – people writing a book and looking for useful material. (The mothers knew they had a story worth telling.) When this role transition took place, the nature of the accounts tended to change. The informants became more relaxed. The conversation became more general and it was easier to probe for detail not immediately relevant to the question of mental handicap. On the other hand, the informants were often less precise and less analytic in stating what they had experienced and what they felt they needed.

A problem with accounts, which you need to look out for in evaluating published research of this kind, is that we all have many different ways of accounting for ourselves, many different stories to tell. There are, for instance, public '**rhetorics**' which people tend to produce in a rounded, rehearsed form when asked direct questions. Some of them are minimal, polite, 'safe', problem-avoiding accounts, what Cornwell (1984) calls 'public accounts': something uncontroversial which is always safe to produce when questioned on this topic. Others are learned rhetorics: the first response on the subject of social class from anyone who has studied sociology, for instance, tends to recapitulate some part of the course studied. Others again are 'class-markers' – to state certain kinds of beliefs communicates membership of a class or group, or sympathy with it. Others again are just well rehearsed stories, polished and perhaps partly falsified or simplified by frequent telling. All or any of these rhetorics may truly be held as beliefs by the informant, and any or all may be acted out in practice, but the chances are that they are sincerely held but purely verbal beliefs, unconnected in any way to action. One always strives to get underneath these rhetorics, to get the informant analysing his or her own life in a fresh way and producing 'true' accounts. However, one should note that these 'private' accounts are equally a product of a particular social situation – the informant striving to make sense of his or her life in the light of his or her perception of what is relevant and useful for the interviewer – so we cannot treat these as necessarily 'more true' than the rhetorics and polished stories.

The points which are important here as guidelines for the evaluation of research are:

1 that informants do not 'give interviewers the facts', but work out the purpose of the interview and give accounts that will make sense and be relevant in the context of that purpose;
2 that they are constrained by what they think is acceptable (as well as relevant) to say to different kinds of people, in different kinds of tasks;
3 that we all have accounts of common topics which 'roll easily off the tongue', but we may have other and possibly contradictory things to say about them if one can get behind the rhetoric; and
4 that any given account may be a rhetoric in this sense, but nonetheless not 'rhetorical' – well practised verbal accounts may or may not be accurate descriptions of behaviour and attitudes.

You would expect to find enough reflexive material in a good account of open interviewing to enable you to form some view on these questions: whether the situation partly dictated the response, whether the interviewer has taken a rhetoric for a reality, whether a well practised account, nonetheless, describes a reality of the informant's life. To the extent that such material is not present, you may have to suspend judgement on the credibility of the results – not necessarily to disbelieve them, but to give them less credit than if their validity was well established.

A second question when evaluating the scope of a piece of research – the opposite of the question of how far it can be generalized – is how specific the findings are. In the Abbott and Sapsford (1987b) paper one important question was the extent to which the experiences of those who care for children with learning difficulties are different from those of other mothers (all mothering being, in a sense, a form of community care). For this reason we also interviewed a group of mothers whose children had not been labelled as having learning difficulties and so were able to distinguish the problems of having children with learning difficulties from the problems of having children in general. (Naturally we took pains to pick a **comparison group** as like the mothers of children with learning difficulties as possible, so that where differences were found they were not equally likely to be due to age or class/material circumstances or area of residence.)

It is worth noting that the interviews with the mothers whose children were not labelled as having learning difficulties were far more difficult than those with mothers whose children were so labelled. The mothers of children with learning difficulties 'knew' what they were being interviewed about – they knew that what we had picked out was mothers in their situation. The other mothers had far more difficulty making sense of the situation. There was no obvious 'social problem' which we might be investigating, and they could not see what it was about their situation which made it interesting for us to get them to 'tell their story'. They therefore had great difficulty working out what story to tell. As we said above, the sense which the informant makes of the situation is a key determinant of the accounts which are elicited in interview.

Summary: points for evaluation

1 When reading 'open interview' research, you need to know quite a lot about the interviewer, the situation and the course of the interviews, to judge the validity of the results. **Reactivity** – the production of material in response to loaded questions, or the reshaping of it to suit the expected prejudices of the interviewer – is a particularly strong possibility in this kind of research.

2 One might be suspicious of research reports based on one quick interview with each informant; the likelihood of the interviewer getting beyond the 'rhetoric' or 'public account' is not high (see Cornwell 1984, particularly p. 16).

3 At a more subtle level, you need to work out what sense the informants probably made of the situation, in order to see what they will have perceived as relevant and what they may have omitted or ignored in their accounts.

4 To the extent that there is insufficient reflexive material for you to make these judgements, you do not need to reject the research report entirely, but its conclusions should be handled with some caution.

5 Looking at the 'sample' you should ask yourself how far the results are likely to generalize beyond the immediate informants – of what are these informants typical?

6 You should also ask yourself how specific the results are to the type of person or setting which is being described – to what extent they might be equally true of quite different groups or settings.

> **Exercise 12**
>
> Now re-read the Abbott and Sapsford (1987b) paper in the light of this chapter, bearing in mind the points listed at the end. Note particularly how much extra material we have had to supply in this chapter in order to give you any real insight into the process of the interviews and the ways in which we were typecast by informants. Look back at the questions you thought you would have liked to ask us. How many of them have been answered by the 'extra' material we have provided in this chapter?

Further reading

On children with learning difficulties

Abbott, Pamela and Sapsford, Roger (1986) Diverse reports: caring for mentally handicapped children in the community, *Nursing Times*, 5 March, 47–9.

Bayley, M. (1973) *Mental Handicap and Community Care*. London: Routledge and Kegan Paul.

Glendinning, C. (1983) *Unshared Care: Parents and their Disabled Children*. London: Routledge and Kegan Paul.

Shearer, A. (1972) *A Report on Public and Professional Attitudes towards the Sexual and Emotional Attitudes of Handicapped People*. London: Spastics Society/National Association for Mental Handicap.

Voysey, M. (1975) *A Constant Burden: The Reconstitution of Family Life*. London: Routledge and Kegan Paul.

On 'normal' mothering

Abbott, Pamela and Wallace, Claire (1996) *An Introduction to Sociology: Feminist Perspectives* (2nd edition). London: Routledge.

Backett, K. (1982) *Mothers and Fathers*. London: Macmillan.

Boulton, M. (1983) *On Being a Mother*. London: Tavistock.

Kitzinger, S. (1978) *Women as Mothers*. London: Fontana.

Oakley, A. (1972) *Sex, Gender and Society*. London: Fontana.

Porter, M. (1983) *Home, Work and Class Consciousness*. Manchester: Manchester University Press.

On coping and coping strategies

Davis, F. (1963) *Passage through Crisis: Polio Victims and their Families.* Indianapolis, IN: Bobbs-Merril.

Goffman, E. (1961) *Asylums: Essays on the Social Situation of Mental Patients and Other Inmates.* Harmondsworth: Penguin.

Goffman, E. (1963) *Stigma: The Management of Spoilt Identities.* Harmondsworth: Penguin.

Roth, J. (1963) *Timetables.* Indianapolis, IN: Bobbs-Merril.

READING OBSERVATION RESEARCH

Research paper 1: Kirkham (1983) 'Labouring in the dark' (observation of labour wards)
Research paper 2: Cayne (1995) 'Portfolios: a developmental influence?' (participant research on nurse professional development)
Research paper 3: James (1984) 'A postscript to nursing' (reflexive account of observation research in hospital)
Summary: points for evaluation
Further reading

This chapter deals with interpretative **observation** studies which involve varying degrees of participation; 'systematic' observation is dealt with under the heading of survey research. The chapter is built around three research papers: Mavis Kirkham (1983) 'Labouring in the dark'; Julia Cayne (1995) 'Portfolios: a developmental influence?'; and Nicky James (1984) 'A postscript to nursing'. All three are reprinted, two of them in slightly shortened form, in Abbott and Sapsford (1997), the Reader associated with this text.

> **Exercise 13**
>
> Now would be a good time to read the first of these three, the paper by Mavis Kirkham, 'Labouring in the dark'.

Research paper 1: Kirkham (1983)

Mavis Kirkham's paper deals with the event of giving birth in hospital and the time leading up to it. Her focus of interest is the transmission – or non-transmission – of information from doctors, nurses and midwives to the pregnant woman, about the progress of her imminent delivery and the timescale that may be expected. She is interested in the hierarchical relationship between nurses and midwives, and patients, and the way in which this may in fact impede delivery by failing to reassure patients and not allowing them to draw on their own strengths during the process.

What she did was to sit in on 90 labours in one consultant unit of a northern teaching hospital, take notes of what was said and done, and talk to the women after their babies had been born; she also talked to 85 patients in hospital before confinement. In addition, she observed five home confinements and 18 confinements in a neighbouring GP unit, and she interviewed a number of midwives. Her method was that of open, unstructured, participant observation:

> I wanted to see what issues were important to those involved as shown in their actions and words at the time. Observation was clearly an appropriate method . . . I came to this research as a midwife and a mother. But my observations were guided by those aspects of care in labour which the midwives and mothers I observed showed were important to them. Thus my observations and analysis were 'grounded' (Glaser and Strauss 1967) in the experiences of those observed as shown in their words and actions.
>
> (Kirkham 1983: 86)

The aim is to describe not necessarily a fully **representative** sample of confinements, but at least a sample of **typical** ones: 'These labours were chosen as normal labours, as far as anyone can tell this in advance. I therefore did not observe women with known medical or obstetric abnormalities' (p. 86).

Kirkham describes and illustrates the main tactics she sees the pregnant women using in order to get information. Straightforward questions are, of course, asked, but this is not always a good tactic for gaining information because questions are often deflected or blocked 'in the patient's interests' or 'because she wouldn't really understand'. Another tactic is to make what appears to be a statement, but which has the force of a question – for example:

> Patient: My backside's hurting. It'll be the cut. [*Silence*] . . . It's the episiotomy.
> Sister: It's not an episiotomy. It's a tear. But it hasn't gone anywhere it shouldn't.

Some patients try out statements in the form of jokes:

> Patient: Is there much water?
> Doctor: A normal amount.
> Patient: You imagine buckets!
> Doctor: You've not got that much when you get to term . . .
>
> (p. 90)

Some combine this with what Kirkham calls 'self-denigration':

> Student midwife [SM]: Let's see if the machine is playing silly beggars.
> [*Patient pulls up her gown to show the . . . connection to the monitor.*]
> SM: You're a right flasher, aren't you?
> Patient: And I've got such a wonderful body.
> [*Both laugh. SM listens to fetal heart. Patient asks if she can listen. SM lets her . . .*]
>
> (p. 91)

Passive watching and the active drawing of conclusions is a common tactic here as elsewhere – 'If it was going to be quick they wouldn't have given me Pethidine' – but it is limited by the extent to which what is seen is correctly understood. A certain amount can be gleaned from eavesdropping on teaching sessions, where sisters are instructing student midwives, for instance, but this essentially passive tactic does not lend itself to the patient gaining useful – usable and interpretable – information.

All of this is contrasted with deliveries in GP units and at home. On the GP units, not surrounded by senior medical staff, midwives were freer with information and found it necessary to solicit the patient's cooperation more. Patients giving birth at home tended to demand to know what was going on.

The author concludes that the women on the ward want and need information with which to orient themselves within the process of birth, and that what they receive is generally inadequate. The lack of information very much constrains their choices. A hierarchy of relations, and of control of information, runs from the patient at the bottom through midwives and sisters to doctors. Kirkham observes that the tactics which patients use to elicit information from midwives run remarkably parallel to those which midwives use to elicit information from doctors. She comments in conclusion that an awareness of problems shared by midwife and patient could do much to change midwives' behaviour, which in turn could fundamentally change the patient's experience of labour.

Exercise 14

Now read Julia Cayne (1995) 'Portfolios: a developmental influence?'

Research paper 2: Cayne (1995)

This paper describes **applied research** undertaken as part of the normal work of the researcher – as a nurse tutor in training in a particular unit, she set up a 'learning group' and monitored its progress.

> A situational analysis had demonstrated a need to help staff within an orthopaedic/trauma unit review past and plan future learning. An **action research** project was undertaken to explore two research questions: is the process of portfolio preparation in itself developmental? If so, what factors influence this developmental process?
>
> (Cayne 1995: 395)

The focus of the group was the actual preparation of portfolios – documentation of past learning – as a cooperative effort within the group (including Cayne, the facilitator).

The membership of the group was somewhat 'happenstance'. In principle, Cayne had permission to approach all qualified nurses on the unit, but in practice the vagaries of shift work determined who was on an early shift on Friday mornings and therefore able to participate, and staffing levels on some units proved a further constraint. In the event a group of six was achieved, one from each of four wards plus one from the accident and emergency department and one from the fracture clinic. The first session was structured to establish the 'contract' for the remaining sessions, but the remaining sessions dealt with problems raised by the group members themselves. Data collection was by the keeping of **field notes**, the taping of group sessions, and taped interviews following an exploratory question-naire (**open-ended questions** – see Chapter 6 below). Each individual was given the chance to comment on a written draft of the findings and to require information to be removed if she felt threatened by its inclusion.

The Results section of the paper begins with a description of the way in which the group facilitated reflection on an individual's career to date. This started as what might be termed 'a vague feeling of discomfort': as one participant put it,

> . . . it gives you – really I suppose a chance for reflection over every-thing, to sort of, I don't know, categorize what you have done and what you haven't done, what you need to do. But and, you feel that it ought to come out with, what I need to do now is this. And when you don't come out with anything specific . . . it feels like nothing's achieved.
>
> (p. 399)

Others described how completing their portfolios made them face up to difficulties in their practice and/or question and revise their self-image. One thing brought home to many of the participants was the value of their professional experience, as opposed to the courses they had taken. The researcher's conclusion was that there were indications that portfolio preparation is developmental in its own right but that the small numbers and short duration of the project make it difficult to provide evidence for this conclusion. Factors which affected the process were uncertainty about the validity of 'subjective' information, fear of failure and, on the other hand, the need to explore and comply with new regulations then coming into force.

The tone of the paper is very reflexive throughout, drawing heavily on the researcher's experience and not trying to any great extent to emulate the 'scientific' style adopted by some research reports:

> I have used the first-person pronoun in the writing of this report because I believe it is an ethical imperative to be open about one's own role in the shaping of events in a project such as this. Webb (1992) points out that the third-person pronoun is used in academic writing to convey 'an impression that the ideas being discussed have a neutral, value free, impartial basis [which] is rarely if ever the case'.
>
> (p. 395)

The belief that the researcher is a neutral scientist who can and should remain detached from what he or she is studying is something we shall dis-cuss elsewhere in this book; it is not a position we take ourselves.

Research paper 3: James (1984)

This concern with reflexivity – a sensitivity to the research as itself a social situation and a part of the researcher's biography – is very characteristic of 'open' research. Both authors are quite aware of their own position within the research, and Mavis Kirkham is explicit about how her position may have affected the behaviour of the women she observed:

> I sat during most of the labours level with the patient's head about six feet from her and took constant written notes. The question of the researcher's influence upon the research is raised by this method . . . The people I observed may well have been on their 'best behaviour' because I was observing them.
>
> (Kirkham 1983: 86)

(In the Cayne paper, despite its open stance, we might have expected to find more discussion of how the fact that she was running the groups might have affected what she found; her control of the topic of conversation, and presumably of its timing and routeing as well, would put her in a strong position to direct the outcome, and because of space constraints we have to take a lot of the conclusions on trust. We might also want to consider the extent to which knowing that they were part of a research project may have altered the participants' approach to the developmental task.) We know from Chapter 4, however, that there is more than the discussion of **reactivity** to a proper **reflexive** account. How the researcher is received and what sense the participants make of her are part of the story that needs to be told. We also need, however, to know more about the researcher herself, her theoretical perspectives, her professional expectations – anything which may affect the conduct of the research or the interpretation of the data.

The third paper to be considered in this chapter, Nicky James's (1984) 'A postscript to nursing', is not a report of research results, but an extended reflexive account, written for a book of articles on the research process. James describes what it was like, as a trained nurse, to return to the wards to do research on nursing for a higher degree. It raises many of the special problems (and the strengths) of the open participation method in an acute form.

Exercise 15

You might like to read the paper at this point: Nicky James (1984) 'A postscript to nursing'.

James went in 'labelled' as a researcher and had no role into which she could 'disappear from view'. Whether participant research should be open or **covert** (secret) is much debated. Covert research obviously disturbs what is going on less; if the researcher can pass as a natural member of the scene, then there is no 'researcher identity' to which participants might react. This obviously holds even more where the researcher is a natural participant in the context. (There are problems of detachment here, however;

it is very difficult to stand back from your own real-life involvement.) The disadvantage of covert research is that you tend to be 'stuck' in one part of the field and bound by the limitations of the adopted role: if you have 'become' a nurse, then you cannot also socialize with doctors on equal terms and experience what the patients experience. You are also limited in the number and type of questions you can ask about what is going on before you start looking unnaturally incompetent and ignorant for a true participant. Some might also consider covert research unethical, in that participants are deceived into revealing things about themselves which they might not have chosen to reveal to a researcher and an abuse of relationships is involved.

• Open research has the converse disadvantage, that participants have to make sense of you and will generally try to consider what they do and say because they know it may be recorded. The presence of an explicit researcher may also be uncomfortable for the other participants because it forces them to question aspects of their behaviour which are normally taken for granted and may partially destroy the careful set of 'cognitive defences' which we all set up against the unpleasant or boring aspects of our jobs and our lives in general. To the extent that real involvement is achieved, moreover, the researcher will also acquire some of these defences, and breaking through them into analysis will become a real emotional problem. (This is also a problem for covert researchers, of course – sometimes more so.) James certainly found both problems during her research relationships with other nurses:

> A dysfunction built into the research . . . was the constant prodding at the defence mechanisms which are a means of continuing at the unit. If I pushed the others too far they would evade, avoid or tell me to shut up, but my own defences were also under scrutiny and the more I was perturbed by exposing them, the more my reluctance to write up at the end of the day grew. I was enjoying the nursing. For the research, philosophy, the structure of the National Health Service, and numbers became easier lines of thought. None of them had anything to do with people.
>
> (James 1984: 141–2)

One of the major problems of undertaking fieldwork, particularly in the role of 'the researcher', is to establish a role within the setting which is something other than sitting and taking notes. As a qualified nurse, Nicky James found it particularly difficult to be present on a ward for which she had no nursing responsibilities, as her field notes show:

> I didn't know what I was doing, and the lack of routine was very undermining, or rather the lack of knowledge of the routine . . . I felt that I had no independence on the ward because I nearly always had to ask people if I wanted to do, or thought I ought to do, something.
>
> (pp. 136–7)

> Confusion and doubt is part of any nurse's move to a new ward, but I had forgotten that and I found it difficult to make sense of things as a nurse, let alone a researcher.
>
> (p. 137)

Having acquired a role within the ward, she found it almost equally difficult to dissociate herself from it again.

The problem for the participants is making sense of the researcher and assigning her a social role, and some of the solutions may not always be flattering or even useful, as James points out:

> Nicky, you're sort of like a PS in a letter. Not part of the main body of the nursing team, but still important.
>
> (Night nurse)

> This is our pet sociologist, who's working on the unit and studying us. She's found out all sorts of interesting things.
>
> (Continuing care unit sister) (p. 129)

What sense will be made is essentially unpredictable, so one has to be prepared to make changes 'on the run'. James had this problem right from the start, in her initial discussions with 'gatekeepers':

> In the proposal to the nursing administrators, submitted before I went to see them, I tried to 'sell' myself by predicting what they would like . . . my main doubt was whether they would tolerate an observer. Why should they? To try to overcome that, I made a commitment to working free, instead of being an onlooker . . . I had totally misjudged their reading of the proposal. Instead of being flexible, it looked as though I did not know what I was doing, and though they welcomed nursing research, there was some anxiety over someone who wanted to be integrated . . . I acquiesced to their suggestions . . . In the report on the meeting I noted that 'I went in optimistic and came out feeling like a grilled sardine – small, squashed and hot.'
>
> (pp. 133–4)

In conclusion, James's account of her research reinforces very strongly the importance of reflexivity. She describes how difficult it was to 'get in' with any freedom of movement, how difficult it was to find herself a role which was plausible to herself, and how difficult it was for others to find a place for her in their social world. She makes it clear that observing was not a neutral process, but one which trampled over her own preconceptions and led to considerable emotional turmoil, the more so because her investigations also tended to trample over the preconceptions and defences of others.

Summary: points for evaluation

1 Observation research, like open interviewing, needs to show a substantial reflexive element in the report if we are to be able to judge the effect of researcher and situation on the recorded data, and how the way in which both researcher and participants make sense of the situation affects what is produced.

2 In observation research even more than in open interviewing we need to know something of the researcher and his or her preconceptions, fears and capabilities, to put faith in the reported interpretations of the situation.

3 In covert research we need to know what kind of role the researcher took up, how convincing he or she was, and the extent to which the role may have tied him or her down to one segment or aspect of the situation and perhaps blinded him or her to interpretations which might seem **valid** from a different perspective. A common criticism of male studies of youth gangs, for instance, is that young women are 'seen' only through the eyes of young men and the male researcher.

4 In research where the researcher is a 'real' participant, carrying out his or her normal role as well as writing about the situation, we need to consider the extent to which it has been possible for him or her to step outside the professional assumptions of that situation for the purposes of the research analysis.

Exercise 16

Now re-read the papers by Kirkham and Cayne in the light of the James paper and our discussion.

Further reading

On maternity nursing

Cartwright, A. (1979) *The Dignity of Labour?* London: Tavistock.

Lorenson, Margarethe (1983) Effects of touch in patients during a crisis situation in hospital, in J. Wilson-Barnett (ed.) *Nursing Research: Ten Studies in Patient Care*. Chichester: Wiley.

Maternity Services Advisory Committee (1984) *Maternity Care in Action Pt II: Care during Childbirth*. London: HMSO.

Maternity Services Advisory Committee (1985) *Maternity Care in Action Pt III: Care of the Mother and Baby*. London: HMSO.

Metcalf, Clare (1983) A study of change in the method of organising the delivery of nursing care in a ward of a maternity hospital, in J. Wilson-Barnett (ed.) *Nursing Research: Ten Studies in Patient Care*. Chichester: Wiley.

Oakley, Ann (1980) *Women Confined: Towards a Sociology of Childbirth*. Oxford: Martin Robertson.

Oakley, Ann (1981) *From Here to Maternity*. Harmondsworth: Penguin.

Savage, Wendy (1986) *A Savage Enquiry: Who Controls Childbirth?* London: Virago.

Developmental learning for professionals

Barber, P. (1989) Developing the 'person' of the professional carer, in S. Hinchcliffe, S. Norman and J. Schober (eds) *Nursing Practice and Health Care*. Sevenoaks: Edward Arnold.

Brookfield, S. (1986) *Understanding and Facilitating Adult Learning*. Milton Keynes: Open University Press.

Rogers, A. (1992) *Adults Learning for Development*. London: Cassell.

Schön, D. (1987) *Educating the Reflective Practitioner*. San Francisco, CA: Jossey-Bass.

Research on general ward nursing

Brown, Roswyn (1989) *Individualised Care: The Role of the Ward Sister*. Harrow: Scutari.

Cope, David (1981) *Organisational Development and Action Research in Hospitals*. Aldershot: Gower.

Wilson-Barnett, Jenifer and Robinson, Sarah (eds) (1989) *Directions in Nursing Research*. Harrow: Scutari.

READING ABOUT CONTROLLED TRIALS

Research paper 1: Gordon (1986) 'Treatment of depressed women by nurses in Britain'
Research paper 2: Doll and Hill (1954) 'The mortality of doctors in relation to their smoking habits'
Summary: points for evaluation
Further reading

At the other extreme of the spectrum of research from open interviewing and observation comes the controlled trial or experiment. The central principle here is not finding out about the unknown, but testing known principles. The medical controlled trial tests the efficacy of a drug or treatment by applying the drug to one group of people and withholding it from another. To the extent that the first group are *exactly* like the second in terms of personal characteristics and histories, and to the extent that they receive *exactly* the same treatment in all ways except that the drug is administered to the experimental group and withheld from the control group, then logically any difference between the two which is present at the end but was not present at the start must be due to the administration of the drug. The four essentials are: a clearly defined 'treatment'; a clearly defined 'outcome'; a comparison of outcomes between treatment and non-treatment, or between different treatments; and control of anything else which might otherwise have explained observed differences in outcome.

Generally, we associate experimental research with highly scientific subject areas – medicine, the more scientific kinds of psychology, etc. It is quite possible, however, to apply precisely the same principles to much more 'woolly' topic areas, such as the treatment of mental conditions; the first paper considered in this chapter is the evaluation of an experimental nurse-administered treatment for women's depression – Verona Gordon's 'Treatment of depressed women by nurses in Britain'.

Exercise 17

You might now like to read the paper by Verona Gordon (1986). The full text, entitled 'Treatment of depressed women by nurses in Britain and the USA', can be found in Julia Brooking (ed.) *Psychiatric Nursing Research*, published by Wiley. A shortened version which omits the USA material will be found in Abbott and Sapsford (1997).

Research paper 1: Gordon (1986)

Verona Gordon's paper begins with a discussion of the extent to which depression can be considered one of the major health problems of women. Twice as many women as men are diagnosed depressed around the world and the incidence of the condition shows an alarming growth over time. (Whether an increased incidence of *diagnosis* of depression over time necessarily equates with an increased *incidence* of depression is questionable, however. We shall return to this point in a later chapter.)

Gordon suggests that current treatment practices are not satisfactory for women's depression:

> There are two concerns that remain with treatment and prevention issues. One is that traditional treatment approaches by male therapists perpetuate the passivity and negative self-image of women . . . The other is that while there are numerous programmes to treat depression, treatment usually begins after the depression has reached a serious level. This lack of early identification and intervention does not support nursing's commitment to prevention and health maintenance.
>
> (Gordon 1986: 95)

She suggests that a group approach is far superior to individual therapy for women, in that it allows for peer support and gives a safe and rewarding environment within which negative self-labelling can be unlearned. The (female) professional nurse, she suggests, is uniquely well placed to run such groups successfully: she is herself a woman (though possibly better educated than some of those she serves); she appreciates the problems of women's positions and the value to them of both family and work; she is not seen by the public as having a judgemental or diagnostic role; and she is popularly stereotyped as someone who cares and offers support.

This paper reports on an experimental treatment group for women's depression which Gordon set up in England. (Two earlier studies were carried out in the United States – see Gordon 1982; Gordon and Ledray 1984).

> Twenty women, 40 to 60 years of age, were selected for the study. These subjects had been recruited through a public service radio broadcast (BBC airwaves) seeking depressed women as participants . . . There was an overwhelming response to the broadcast from hundreds of women . . . The University of London's phone lines were flooded with calls, confirming the author's belief that depression in women is extensive.
>
> (p. 100)

'Information meetings' were set up, at which 119 women who showed interest and met the criteria filled out a descriptive questionnaire and took two standardized tests of depression and suicidal pathology. Eighty-one women showed up on these tests as mildly to moderately depressed, and 20 of these were randomly selected for the treatment group. A similar-sized group of women were selected from the 81 as a control group, and they filled in the same tests as these 20 at around the same time. However, women assigned to the control condition received no intervention between pre- and post-testing. At the first information meeting they had been asked to refrain from joining other therapy groups or seeking counselling while the study was going on unless necessary.

(p. 105)

(The women who were not to be used in the study were, nonetheless, informed of their test results by post. Gordon telephoned the six who showed up as very depressed; all of them agreed to consult their GP.)

Meetings were arranged for the 20 women in a comfortable central location in London, and the discussion group began to meet. In the first meetings all the women were encouraged to 'tell their story', but subsequently such working over past ground was discouraged. Instead, a topic was assigned for each meeting – signs and symptoms of depression, assertiveness, goal-setting, conflict management, etc. – and this was discussed, with Gordon introducing educational material into the discussion. Homework tasks were set and a workbook issued. At the start of the series of meetings, all subjects filled in five self-report tests, all of proven reliability and widely used in research, covering self-esteem, social adjustment, loneliness, depression/hopelessness and 'life events' occurring. The same tests were re-administered at the end of the 14 group sessions.

The results were fairly clear-cut. There were no significant pre-treatment differences between the experimental group and the controls. Three of the tests – depression, self-esteem and hopelessness – showed significant post-test differences between the experimental group and the control group. *Prima facie* the results suggest strongly that the treatment made a difference to the attitudes and internal states of those who received it.

The author's conclusions are:

1 that professional nurses . . . tend to be effective facilitators of depressed women's groups;
2 that coping strategies for women can be taught, tested and shared within a supportive group atmosphere;
3 that replication of the intervention model with increased numbers of women of a variety of ages and backgrounds could be useful future nursing research.

The significance of the intervention model is:

1 to help women cope effectively and take an active role in their own health;
2 to prevent possible severe depression in women;
3 to gain data about the complex phenomena of depression in women;
4 to strengthen the family unit by increasing self-esteem of women.

(pp. 112–13)

(The first conclusion is possibly stronger than the design of the study warrants: one may not conclude that 'nurses tend' on the basis of results from one or a few nurses. The best that can be said is that nurses *are able* to act as facilitators.)

As an example of a 'controlled trial', this experiment in therapy shows many of the classic features of the true experiment as used in medicine or psychology, but falls down in some respects and is questionable in others. (This is not a criticism of the particular study, but the general verdict on the use of this research approach to evaluate events which happen outside the 'pure science' laboratory.) Its strength is in the clean lines of its design – a treatment applied to one group and withheld from another, with demonstrably little pre-treatment difference between the groups and demonstrably significant differences after the treatment. (The concept of 'significance' will be dealt with in a later chapter. For now, accept as a suitable simplification that a result is described as 'significant' if the odds against it occurring by chance are very high.)

There are two questions which might sensibly be asked of this as an experiment, however, issues on which it perhaps fails to reach the rigour of the 'true' laboratory experiment or hospital controlled trial.

1 The 'manipulation' is somewhat vaguely defined. If someone were to try to duplicate the procedures and obtained the opposite effect we would not know whether this argued against Gordon's findings or merely demonstrated that the new researcher had not, in fact, managed to duplicate Gordon's procedures. This is a general point about the evaluation of therapies.
2 The second potential criticism concerns the measure of outcome – the questionnaires which the subjects filled in. At least in this study we have what purports to be an objective measure of outcome – as opposed to therapist's or patient's judgement, which are obviously suspect in this context. However, this fact that the 'measures' are predesigned questionnaires purporting to give a score for some predetermined mental trait, state or circumstance is always a reason for pausing to think about the research. We shall discuss such measures in the next chapter and elsewhere in the book. You might want to ask yourself, however, the extent to which you could realistically expect any kind of prestructured questionnaire to reflect people's real experience of the complex, social phenomenon which we call depression. (Note, however, that this criticism does not necessarily hold true for the test used to select the experimental and control groups. These did not purport to explain/describe depression, but merely to predict whether it was likely to occur, and even an ill-theorized test can turn out empirically to have considerable predictive value.)

Research paper 2: Doll and Hill (1954)

For the second paper in this chapter we go back 30 years, to a classic of health research. A number of studies (among them Doll and Hill 1950) had demonstrated that there were fewer non-smokers among patients with lung cancer and more heavy smokers than among patients suffering from other diseases. This kind of comparison has some of the structure of an experiment: if we think of cancer patients as the 'experimental' group and other patients as the 'controls', it would appear that there is an association between smoking and the likelihood of becoming a cancer patient. The temptation is to go beyond asserting just an *association*, to the supposition that it may be smoking that causes cancer (or at least *some* cancer): we have a prior factor – smoking – and a subsequent variation in incidence of cancer, so it seems not unreasonable that the cancer may be consequent on the smoking. The logic is weaker than that of the true experiment, however, because so many *other* differences could also have an effect. People who smoke may differ from people who do not smoke in any number of ways: personally they could be more anxious and tense, for example, or as a group they might tend to be in different kinds of occupations which put them into a higher risk category, or smokers might tend to be older on average than non-smokers, or there might be any number of other differences which might be responsible for the difference in cancer incidence.

Some of these had been eliminated by collecting data on them in the original survey. In their 1950 paper, for example, Doll and Hill were able to look at the gender, age and social class of cancer patients and non-cancer patients; the two groups did not differ in age or gender, so these are not likely to be causal factors (but there *were* some minor differences in social class, and quite large differences in place of residence). Another way of dealing with differences, if any had been found, would have been by statistical control: comparisons can be made in ways which are not affected by known differences on other variables. For example, it would have been possible to compare cancer rates among younger people, separately from older ones, and so do away with the effect of age on any perceived differences. Nonetheless, logical doubts must remain; we cannot control for everything – and certainly not for factors on which it has not occurred to us to collect information. Further, there is always the possibility that something about the situation leads to higher reporting (in this case of smoking) in one group than the other, or that something in the research procedures made a cancer patient's smoking more likely to be recorded.

> Another possibility to consider is that the lung-carcinoma patients tended to exaggerate their smoking habits . . . they would have known that they had respiratory symptoms, and such knowledge might have influenced their replies to questions about the amount they smoked . . . consideration must [also] . . . be given to the possibility of interviewer bias affecting the results (by the interviewers tending to scale up the smoking habits of the lung-carcinoma patients).
>
> (Doll and Hill 1950: 745)

The second of these was controlled, in the 1950 study, by looking at those cases thought to be cancerous at the time of interview whose diagnosis was subsequently changed, and they did not appear to have their smoking in any way exaggerated by the interviewers. The first can be argued against on the basis of other patients with respiratory diseases, who did not appear in the 1950 study to differ in their smoking habits from patients with other kinds of illness. Nonetheless some doubt must remain, and a different kind of study was needed.

> **Exercise 18**
>
> You may now like to read the paper – Richard Doll and A. Bradford Hill (1954) 'The mortality of doctors in relation to their smoking habits', in *British Medical Journal* (26 June, pp. 1451–5). It is also reprinted in Abbott and Sapsford (1997).

This study is a *prospective survey* in design: it identifies groups of people who differ in some respect and follows them up to see the outcome of their differences. In this case the researchers wrote to every member of the UK medical profession in October 1951 and asked them to fill in a short questionnaire giving name, address, age, and 'smoking behaviour' – whether they were current smokers, had smoked in the past but since given up, or had never smoked regularly (defined as 'as much as one cigarette per day or its equivalent in pipe tobacco for as long as a year'). Current smokers were asked the age at which they started smoking and the method of smoking, and ex-smokers were asked similar questions relating to the time immediately prior to giving up. Nearly 60,000 questionnaires were sent out, and about 41,000 were returned, of which 40,564 were sufficiently complete to be usable. (This gives a usable response rate of 68 per cent – in other words, the returned and usable forms covered two-thirds of the doctors in the UK.) Lung cancer is relatively rare in men younger than 35 and in women, however, so these forms were discarded, leaving 26,389 forms for analysis.

From the replies the doctors were classified into broad groups by age, amount of smoking, method of smoking and whether they were current smokers or had given up. Additional information was collected from the Registrar General for the United Kingdom – a form showing particulars of death for every doctor who had died since completing the questionnaire. Thirty-six deaths certified as from lung cancer were discovered in this way; checking on the evidence for the diagnosis by writing to the doctors who had signed the death certificates they found that 'there were firm grounds for the diagnosis in at least 33 of the cases, and in only three was the evidence limited to clinical examination'. Deaths from other cancers, respiratory diseases, coronary thrombosis, other cardiovascular diseases and 'other diseases' were also recorded. A total of 789 deaths occurred among the group in the 29 months after the questionnaire was sent out.

Death rates differed very markedly between smokers and non-smokers. No non-smokers died of lung cancer during the period, for example, but 0.48 men per thousand of the light smokers (i.e. about one man in 2000 in this category), 0.67 per thousand of medium smokers and 1.14 per thousand of heavy smokers died of lung cancer; in other words, the death rate for this disease was well over twice as high for heavy smokers as for light smokers, and immeasurably smaller for non-smokers. Differences for coronary thrombosis showed a similar but less marked pattern. Deaths from the other diseases did not show this pattern at all; for example, death rates from other cancers were *higher* for non-smokers than for smokers.

It was noted, however, that smoking habits varied considerably with age and that cancer incidence also varied with age, so age could be an

Table 5.1   Actual and expected lung-cancer deaths in the Doll and Hill research

	Non-smokers	Smokers		
		Light	Average	Heavy
Actual deaths	0	12	11	13
Expected deaths	3.77	14.20	10.73	7.33

Source: Doll and Hill (1954: 1453).

alternative explanation of the results: perhaps age was responsible for the cancer, and also responsible independently of the cancer for the amount people smoke. This was examined in the 1954 paper by calculating the number of deaths from lung cancer that would be expected in each age band separately, irrespective of smoking level, and thence how many deaths there ought to have been among light, average, heavy and non-smokers if the number of deaths were independent of the amount smoked. The results are shown in Table 5.1, and it can be seen that we would have expected four deaths among the non-smokers but in reality there were none. Fourteen deaths would have been expected among the light smokers and only seven among the heavy smokers, but the actual figures were 12 and 13 respectively – many more deaths in the 'heavy smoking' category than would have been expected on the basis of age alone.

As you can see, the data-collection design of a survey like this is relatively simple compared with the design of an experiment – you just send out questionnaires and hope to get a reasonably high proportion back usefully filled in. *After* data collection, however, a lot is done in analysis to try to emulate the logic of comparison which is built into the design of a true experiment. The 'treatment group' is smokers (a self-administered treatment!), and the control or comparison group is non-smokers. An apparent effect of smoking is demonstrated – smokers are much more likely than non-smokers to die of lung cancer, even over the relatively short period of the study (29 months) – and the likelihood of smoking being the causal factor is increased by the fact that the lung-cancer death rate increases with the *amount* smoked. This is only the start of the analysis, however; much remains to be done, to eliminate alternative plausible explanations for the results.

Some of them are eliminated in this study at the design stage, by the choice of respondents. One problem with the retrospective studies discussed earlier was that the possibility that the control group was selected in a biased fashion because the nature of the study was known, and another was the possibility that those who knew they had lung cancer might have exaggerated the amount they smoked in the light of this knowledge. The first of these possibilities is eliminated in the 1954 study by the fact that the control group is not selected by the researchers but given 'in nature': we compare people who smoke with people who have not smoked. The second is eliminated by the prospective nature of the study; at the time when the level of smoking is being reported, none of the deaths has occurred. A third problem with the retrospective study, that likelihood of dying of lung cancer was associated with occupation, is eliminated in this study by using only doctors as respondents, and further distracting possibilities are eliminated by discarding the women and those under the age of 35 from the sample.

Because the allocation to 'experimental' or 'control' group is not under the control of the researcher and not conducted randomly, however, other possibilities arise which have to be eliminated in the analysis. For example, because the groups are not of equal sizes we cannot just compare raw numbers of deaths; we have to express the deaths as rates per thousand or percentages to eliminate the effect of unequal group size. It was also noticed that lung-cancer death rate and level of smoking both varied with age, so age was a possible cause of both (independently of each other). This was eliminated as a plausible alternative explanation, however, by calculating 'expected numbers' on the basis of age alone, irrespective of smoking level, and showing that amount smoked had an effect on the death rate over and above what would be expected on the basis of age alone.

A second point we might reasonably make is that real answers often take more than a single study to produce. We often talk as if the 'unit of research' were the experiment or the survey or the set of interviews, but quite often it makes better sense to talk about a whole *programme* of research. In the case of the lung-cancer research, an initial study confirmed earlier work and showed that there was an apparent association between smoking and lung cancer – in other words, that there *was* a question to answer. It also cleared up one or two of the possible alternative explanations – age and gender, for example. Considering possible objections in terms of the methods of the study – possible reactive effects of the situation on the answers given, or possible unconscious biases in the interviewers – the authors were able to deal with some, but others were inherent in the design of the study. The 1954 paper has a different, prospective design – it collects data on people who do not yet have the cancer, and then waits to see which of them contract it – which avoids many of the methodological problems of the earlier work. Further alternative explanations are dealt with: social class (or rather, something associated with it, such as working conditions) is not the causal factor, because the differences hold up when we consider people who are all in the same profession. A second report of the prospective study (Doll and Hill 1956) confirms the trends, with more certainty because the number of deaths concerned was (obviously) greater after four years than only 29 months. It also deals with whether place of residence is a causal factor (e.g. because of atmospheric pollution) and shows that the effect holds in remote rural areas as well as in the inner cities, so this is eliminated as an alternative explanation of the results. In a final report the analysis is repeated in more detail, with a still larger sample of deaths. The authors had also sent a follow-up questionnaire to surviving doctors in the interim, asking whether their smoking habits had changed, and so they were able to show in the 1960 paper that death rates among those who continued to smoke during the whole period of the study were significantly higher than among those who stopped smoking in the course of it.

This programme is a good example of what we sometimes call quasi-experimental analysis – a comparison like an experiment in form, and following the same logic as an experiment, but not truly experimental because the independent variable (the one which is supposed to have a causal effect) is not under the control of the researcher. In this case the dependent variable is death from lung cancer and the proposed independent (causal) variable is smoking – whether the subject smokes at all, and the *amount* he smokes if so. A connection is easily demonstrated, but there are many possible alternative explanations for it which might be advanced, to do with other variables on which those who died differed from those who did not or to do with the way in which the research was carried out. The papers we have discussed constitute a systematic, careful and painstaking attempt to eliminate each of these alternative explanations in order to show that the smoking was not itself caused by a variable which also caused the cancer. It is this kind of programme which most evidently demonstrates the point we made earlier, that any research report travels from a problem to a conclusion supported by evidence, *via* a series of arguments as to why the evidence should be taken to mean what the researchers say it means.

One more point to note is that in many experiments and quasi-experiments the outcome measure is more trivial, more artificial, less 'real and earnest', than the real thing for which it is taken as proxy. This is not the case in the Doll and Hill research – the dependent variable is death from cancer, not some more trivial substitute. (In general, one advantage of quasi-experimental analysis is that it makes research possible on real-life topics where true experiments could not be carried out for ethical or practical reasons.) However, even so it is not a perfect operationalization of what the authors want to study. Their interests are in what causes cancer; their research, for reasons of accessibility of data, is on *deaths* from cancer, which is not quite the same thing.

(You will find, incidentally, that what this kind of research is *called* varies according to the discipline from which the research emanates. In social research, studies which involve a controlled manipulation by the researcher are called 'experiments', while studies which depend on comparing naturally occurring cases are called 'quasi-experiments' or a kind of 'survey'. In medical and health research the former is often called a 'controlled trial' if it involves the testing of a drug or procedure, while studies comparing, for instance, otherwise similar people who do or do not have a given disease are referred to as 'case-control studies'.)

Summary: points for evaluation

1 Controlled trials, experiments and studies which are like experiments stand or fall by two factors: (a) clear definition and measurement of a dependent variable (the thing to be influenced) and one or more independent variables (the thing(s) doing the influencing); (b) the elimination of all other possible explanations of any obtained changes in the dependent variable.

2 In quasi-experimental analysis ('case-control studies') both of these are likely to be problematic, but the researchers should do their best to convince us that other plausible explanations are ruled out.

3 The major way in which change is demonstrated – and a large class of other explanations eliminated – is by comparison between groups which differ on the independent variable. The comparison is often based on a contrast between an 'experimental' group which receives some treatment and a 'control' group from whom it is withheld. The logic of the argument will work only to the extent that these groups are comparable.

4 In some studies a 'same subjects' design will be used, with the same person participating, sequentially, in the 'experimental' and the 'control' condition. In this case, however, it is important to rule out explanations of observed changes in terms of changes in the people concerned – learning, fatigue, etc.

5 However perfect the design, experimental research very often suffers from a tendency to trivialize or 'artificialize' the real situation which it is seeking to simulate. This should be looked out for in evaluating such studies.

Exercise 19

Now re-read the two papers in the light of our comments.

Further reading

Women and psychiatry

Brown, George and Harris, Tirril (1978) *Social Origins of Depression: A Study of Psychiatric Disorder in Women*. London: Routledge and Kegan Paul.
Busfield, Joan (1991) *Women and Mental Health*. London: Macmillan.
Fulani, Lenora (ed.) (1988) *The Politics of Race and Gender in Therapy*. New York: Haworth Press.
Nairn, K. and Smith, G. (1984) *Dealing with Depression*. London: Women's Press.
Orr, Jean (ed.) (1986) *Women's Health in the Community*. Chichester: Wiley.
Penfold, Susan and Walker, Gillian (1984) *Women and the Psychiatric Paradox*. Milton Keynes: Open University Press.

Smoking and lung cancer

Ashton, Heather and Stepney, Rob (1982) *Smoking: Psychology and Pharmacology*. London: Tavistock.
Graham, Hilary (1993) *When Life's a Drag: Smoking and Disadvantage*. London: HMSO.
Doll, Richard and Peto, Richard (1981) *The Causes of Cancer: Quantitative Estimates of Avoidable Risks of Cancer*. Oxford: Oxford University Press.

READING SURVEY RESEARCH

Research paper 1: Abbott (1997) 'Home helps and district nurses: community care in the far South West'
Research paper 2: Abbott and Sapsford (1993) 'Studying policy and practice: use of vignettes'
Discussion
Summary: points for evaluation
Further reading

Surveys are about finding out what is there – asking questions or observing, and counting the answers. (This is far too simple a definition to encompass anything like the full range of survey research, as we shall quickly see, but it is a good starting point.) The 'ideal survey' is the 10-yearly **Census** of Population, when squads of interviewers (known as enumerators) receive standardized training and then go out to find every household in the country and get the answers to a range of basic questions about the people living there. Most surveys are smaller in scale than this and cannot hope to reach every member of the population. What they do is to ask questions of a *sample* of the population and hope that this sample is **representative** – that what is true of the sample will be true of the population as a whole. The General Household Survey, for instance, is another large government survey, happening more frequently than the Census, which also asks for household composition and living standards, but of a **randomly** drawn sample of the population – quite a large sample, but only a small percentage of the people who might have been asked. If the sample is random and reasonably large, then we can have every confidence that it is reasonably representative.

Most surveys are smaller still – including the one at which we shall look in this chapter. They share two key issues with larger ones, however. The first is the question of representation: to the extent that a survey sets out to describe a population on the basis of a sample, it has to be able to demonstrate that the sample is likely to be representative of that population. The second is **validity of measurement**: the answers, which are ultimately recorded as numerical codes, have to have been produced by clear, appropriate questions, or 'measuring instruments', which really do measure what the researcher says they measure.

The example examined in this chapter consists of two research papers describing a project carried out in Cornwall into the provision of community care to older and/or disabled people by home helps and district nurses. The first of the two papers may be seen as primarily descriptive – it examines what services are actually provided and by whom – with the intent of making recommendations about the 'skill mix' needed and how it may best be provided. However, many surveys are not just descriptive. They have a **quasi-experimental** element about them: they were set up to test some statement about differences between two or more groups, or the (**causal**) **association** of two variables. The Doll and Hill paper in the last chapter, which we described there as quasi-experimental, was a survey; all quasi-experimental analyses are also survey based.

Exercise 20

You may now like to read the first of the papers, Pamela Abbott (1997) 'Home helps and district nurses: community care in the far South West', in Abbott and Sapsford (eds) *Research into Practice: A Reader for Nurses and the Caring Professions* (2nd edition).

Research paper 1: Abbott (1997)

This is a much shortened summary of a multi-method project carried out in Cornwall in 1992, which examined community care provision in three GP practices – a small market town, a small coastal port and a village. (The port and the village received district nursing services from the same team, which was based in a nearby small town.) Abbott points out that Cornwall is not **typical** of the rest of the country – no county is entirely typical of any other – in that it has a large elderly population (as a 'retirement area') and faces particular problems of service delivery because of geographical isolation leading to high transport costs both for the service providers and for the old people themselves (coupled, for the latter, with low availability). However, Cornwall faces the same problems of policy and practice in delivering care as other areas, so its practices may illuminate those of other areas also.

The first point made in the paper is that 'community care' is not synonymous with 'statutory services'. Other 'literature' shows that only a very small percentage of those aged 65 or older receive help from the state or voluntary agencies: about 7 per cent attend a day centre or lunch club, about 1 per cent receive 'meals on wheels', and around 4 per cent are clients of the home help or district nursing services. (The figures rise, for those aged 75+, to 7 and 5 per cent for day centres and 'meals on wheels', 8 per cent receive district nursing, and about 14 per cent have a home help.) Most care is provided by relatives, with spouses accounting for about two-thirds of it (the other substantial category being daughters or daughters-in-law) – and it is worth remembering from the start that the vast majority of these spouses were themselves old and perhaps frail.

Fieldwork comprised five elements:

1 a 'casing' of the area – talking to social services and health authority staff and GPs and following up contacts, to identify all the statutory and voluntary services offered to older people and those commercial services

which were discounted for older people (e.g. pubs offering a special price on meals for pensioners);

2 structured interviews with carers and those who were cared for, to identify the services they received and how they felt about them, and to collect some basic demographic information (e.g. age, type of residence, distance from nearest family member);

3 a structured **questionnaire** to home helps and district nurses, to ascertain the services they provided formally and informally, and their attitudes to the work;

4 a structured questionnaire was completed by district nurse team leaders and home help organizers which was designed to elicit information on who was responsible for care tasks for clients in different circumstances;

5 home helps and district nurses were accompanied on their rounds by one of the researchers.

The interview with carers and the 'cared-for' was administered to 100 clients in total – 32 men and 68 women – identified by district nursing team leaders and/or senior home helps as users of their services in the three GP practices in October 1991. (All agreed to take part, but not every client answered every question.) A list of care tasks was derived from the home help and district nurse job descriptions and from common-sense analysis of the needs of older people; the interviewer asked which of these were received on a regular basis, and from whom. 'Informal' carers (relatives, friends, neighbours) provided domestic and social rather than personal and nursing care – shopping was the task most frequently mentioned. Sixty-one informants were being seen by a member of the district nursing team, and 54 had home helps. Home helps most often provided general housework and/or social care tasks (e.g. shopping, accompanying to doctor, collecting pension, paying bills) but also carried out some personal care tasks, the most frequent being helping with bathing. District nurses (or auxiliaries) most frequently gave medical/nursing treatment, help or advice and personal care tasks (bathing, washing, help with getting up or going to bed). There were some discrepancies between what clients said they received and what providers said they provided, but on the whole the answers paralleled each other. While the great majority of district nursing patients required nursing care, all the members of the district nursing team except three said they visited patients requiring only personal care – bathing, shaving or getting up/getting to bed.

A majority of users received only one statutory service, but a small number had more than one. Sometimes this was because a very specialized service was being received (e.g. Macmillan nursing), but sometimes both home helps and district nurses visited the same client. Mostly they provided complementary services, but there was overlap in the provision of personal care (e.g. bathing), particularly in the area in which the district nursing team included auxiliaries.

[I]f we examine the cases where clients were visited by both . . . there seems to be a clear division of tasks. In the majority of cases the interview and observation data suggest that the district nurses were carrying out specialised nursing tasks and the home helps personal care tasks. Observation of the district nurses in [two of the practices] suggests they carry out personal care tasks . . . on days or at times when the home help was not visiting. In [the third practice] . . . most personal care, including baths, was done by home helps. However, the district nurses were concerned about the ability of the home helps to do personal care and the home helps felt that they were not recognised as part of the care team by the district nurses.

(Abbott 1997: 89)

Both district nurses and home helps were asked whether they ever performed tasks for clients which were not on the agreed care plan. All except one of the district nurses admitted to doing so, the tasks frequently mentioned being generally related to nursing care – collecting dressings and prescriptions, making tea/coffee, occasionally making breakfast if the patient was unwell. Other tasks mentioned by at least one included advice on forms, changing light bulbs, washing underwear, lighting the fire and putting dirty linen in to soak. However, few tasks overall were performed which were not part of the nursing care plan. Most of the home helps said clients asked them to do tasks additional to their duties – mostly occasional or heavy cleaning tasks – and nearly all said clients telephoned them at home, to do shopping before they next called or occasionally because they required help (for example, after a fall).

Where district nurses visited patients who were also visited by home helps, most regarded themselves as having regular contact with the home helps, though sometimes only on a casual basis. Most of the home helps had clients whose care was shared with district nurses, and all thought that the arrangements worked well. Liaison was sometimes a problem, however:

Ten of the home helps said that they had opportunity to liaise with the district nurse. One other . . . said there was liaison with a senior. The home helps seemed to feel that they had less opportunity to liaise with the district nurses than vice versa. Observation and information obtained from interviewing would indicate that this liaison was ad hoc and opportunistic rather than formalised.

(Abbott 1997: 92)

District nurses receive the standard nursing training and then do a post-qualification course (though the auxiliaries are not trained nurses and are considered to be under the supervision of a qualified nurse at all times). Home helps said they received very little training for the domestic and personal care tasks they undertake. All except two of the informants said they had done the basic three-day home help course on duties and responsibilities, nutrition and hygiene, incontinence, the lifting of clients, and health and safety aspects of the job. The three senior home helps had also done City and Guilds qualifications. The level and status of work seems to be seen as inferior to that of nurses (or even the relatively untrained auxiliaries) by the district nursing team and the clients – which, of course, makes them seen at the same time as more approachable by clients.

Only one home help expressed a negative view of her work . . . 'Some people call us the Community Dogsbodies'. However, while we were accompanying home helps in two of the areas, a number of them

referred to the negative stereotype that they thought home helps had
. . . and suggested that the district nurses (including auxiliaries) looked
down on them . . . One mentioned a meeting . . . where the auxiliaries
had said that they would not take on the work home helps did because
it was demeaning . . . We were told that clients would not think of
asking nurses to do extra tasks for them or ringing them at home, and
our research appears to bear this out.

(Abbott 1997: 94)

Senior home helps have guaranteed hours of work, but the basic-grade
workers are all employed part-time and have no guaranteed hours of work;
for some, fluctuation in hours was a financial problem. Despite this, and
despite a general feeling that there was too little time to do the job properly
and chat with clients, home helps exhibited a very high level of job satisfaction. In defining their job, most emphasized the caring or helping element, and most felt that the words 'carer' or 'caring' would be appropriate in
the job title. Most said they had joined the service because they wanted to
help people and because it was a job which drew on their skills and experience as carers in the domestic sphere.

> **Exercise 21**
>
> The second paper in this chapter, which you may want to read now, is a
> more detailed report on one aspect of this research – Abbott and
> Sapsford (1993) 'Studying policy and practice: use of vignettes'. This
> was originally published in *Nurse Researcher* (1993) and is reprinted in
> Abbott and Sapsford (eds) (1997), *Research into Practice: A Reader for
> Nurses and the Caring Professions* (2nd edition).

Research paper 2: Abbott and Sapsford (1993)

This paper picks up one particular aspect of the Cornish research and
examines it in more depth. Part of the questionnaire sent to home help
organizers and district nursing team leaders – the people who actually
made assessments of needs in the real situation and allocated services – was
a series of **'vignettes'** on which notional decisions were to be made. A
vignette is a short description or story – a fictional situation – which can be
discussed in the same kind of way as comparable real situations are discussed. Vignettes have the advantage over real-life situations (a) that they
can be discussed without the ethical and practical implications of discussing real cases, while still being closer to real situations than generalized
questions about policy or practice divorced from actual cases, (b) they
allow a range of cases to be covered which is wider than would probably be
encountered in research observing real cases over some finite time-period,
and (c) that the details can be varied systematically to test ideas about the
decisions people make. They have been widely used in social psychology,
in research on decision-making and moral reasoning, and in social policy

research to examine professionals' use of concepts such as 'child abuse' and to measure attitudes to community care. All the home help organizers and district nursing team leaders were sent the questionnaire, and usable replies were received from 19 team organizers and 28 team leaders.

A typical vignette would be 'Case 1: Mr and Mrs Jones':

> Mr and Mrs Jones, who are in their early 70s, live in a modern bungalow about a mile from local shops and ten miles from the nearest town. They both have occupational pensions in addition to the state's. Mrs Jones can drive, but Mr Jones, who has Parkinson's disease, has severe mobility problems and is no longer able to leave the house without professional assistance. He attends the day hospital one day a week and has regular periods of respite care. Mrs Jones has a heart condition and has had two hip replacements – both of which are now causing her problems. They moved to Cornwall on retirement and have no relatives living locally.

Respondents were asked to say who should be providing help with a range of tasks (e.g. bathing, shaving, treating pressure areas, shopping, housework), from a long list of possible providers (including spouse, friends, neighbours and relatives as well as 'professional' providers). In the paper we consider how the responses have been clustered, in order to examine a 'skills mix' question, into 'district nurse', 'home help', 'both', 'neighbour/friend' and 'relation' – the last category including spouse. The results are summarized in Table 6.1 for six of the tasks.

Even in this small sample of responses some pattern can be seen. Nursing care (exemplified here by 'treating pressure areas') is seen as a nursing

Table 6.1 Responses to Vignette 1 in the Cornish research for six selected tasks (%)

Task	District nurse and home help	District nurse alone	Home help alone	Neigh-bour/ friend	Relative
Home help organizer responses					
Bathing Mr Jones	44	17	28	—	—
Shaving Mr Jones	6	—	88	—	6
Treating pressure areas	17	78	—	—	—
Shopping	—	—	78	6	17
Meal preparation	—	—	44	—	38
Light housework	—	—	28	—	22
District nurse team leader responses					
Bathing Mr Jones	22	48	22	—	—
Shaving Mr Jones	30	7	52	—	11
Treating pressure areas	26	70	4	—	—
Shopping	—	—	79	17	4
Meal preparation	—	—	74	7	11
Light housework	—	—	64	—	18

Note: Percentages in some rows total less than 100 because of missing answers or 'other' responses.

province, as one would expect, though some respondents thought home helps could also administer the treatment, alone or in conjunction with district nurses (only the nursing team leaders suggesting home helps alone). Personal care – bathing, shaving – is seen as the province of both home helps and district nurses; home help organizers were most likely to suggest a combination of the two for bathing, and were relatively unlikely to suggest district nurses on their own. Shaving, however, was seen as overwhelmingly a home help task. Nursing team leaders see a larger role for district nurses in personal care – particularly bathing – but over half relegated shaving to the home helps. Shopping, meal preparation and housework are seen as home help jobs and not appropriate for district nurses, but the spouse is also expected to play a part, particularly by the home help organizers. Other small insights may be gleaned which would be worth following up. For example, although no neighbours are mentioned in the vignette, and indeed it is suggested that the house may be quite isolated, a small proportion of home help organizers thought neighbours should do the shopping (and quite a large proportion of nursing team leaders), and a small proportion of nursing team leaders thought they should help with cooking.

Overall, for a wide range of different kinds of 'case', there was substantial agreement among respondents both within and between respondents that nursing tasks belonged predominantly to district nurses and domestic ones to home helps. Home helps were sometimes seen as appropriate for the former (after training, presumably), but district nurses were never seen as appropriate for the latter. There were some differences as regards personal care, mostly in the direction of district nurse team leaders tending to see this more as a part of nursing than did home help organizers. There were also interesting differences in the extent to which spouses (particularly wives) and relatives living within reasonable reach are seen as responsible for domestic, social and (if female) personal care. Thus in this paper the vignette technique has enabled the researchers to explore a wide range of different kinds of 'community care problem' and obtain detailed information on concrete cases, avoiding the **rhetoric** of generalized questions and the ethical and practical difficulties of scrutiny of real cases.

Discussion

Three points are worth considering about these papers and all others of their kind, points which bear directly on our evaluation of published research. The first is the question of measurement. As we noted earlier, clear measurement of the quantities which are to be counted is quite essential for this kind of research. The structured Cornish research questionnaires, asking for a list of the services which are performed or received, come off quite well in this respect; the questions which were asked were obviously quite clear and 'factual'. However, we should note the discrepancies between professionals' accounts of what they provide and users' accounts of what they receive. These may be due to poor memory, but they may also be due to lack of knowledge – where district nurses claim to be giving far more advice than users claim to be receiving, for example, they may not realize that what the researchers mean by 'advice' includes casual chats and incidental suggestions. If this explains the difference, then we would describe it as being an artefact produced by **reactivity** – produced by differential interpretation of the questions rather than by the practice which the questionnaire is intended to measure, and so a product of the design of the questionnaire rather than of the social situation at which it is aimed. Secondly, on the other hand, the difference may be seen as a real one, between the world-pictures of the professionals and the users – that the professionals (deliberately) proffer advice in forms in which it will not be seen as advice by the users – in which case both could be 'right' about what goes on. A third possibility is that the discrepancy is due simply to faulty memory on the part of one party or the other. This is less likely in this case, where the events and practices under examination are relatively recent. Longer-term questions, about events which have happened in the more distant past, would be more suspect in this respect. Memory of the past is prone to inflation or diminution, depending on what point the informant thinks the survey is trying to prove. In survey research, just as much as in less structured styles, the informant makes sense of the situation and tailors his or her replies accordingly.

Even within these structured questionnaires, however, some of the questions should not be taken as simply factual – those on 'how you feel about . . .' some aspect of the situation. How do you feel about reading this book, at this precise moment? Are you satisfied? Fairly satisfied? Neither satisfied nor unsatisfied? Puzzled about how to answer the question, given that some aspects of the book may be quite useful, but others are clearly tedious or over-simple? Puzzled about how to answer the question before you have finished reading it and had time to think about it and perhaps use it in other contexts?

The vignette measurements certainly need more thought and justification, because they concern not what *is* done but what *should* be done or *would* be done, in a hypothetical situation. This raises a second aspect of reactivity – the artificiality of the situation and the extent to which what is produced by respondents is a reaction to that artificial situation and fails to generalize to 'real' life beyond it. (A frequent criticism of 'scientific' social psychology, for example, is that it has spent over a century working out the rules and laws of social behaviour in artificial small groups, in laboratories, and is still no nearer to explaining what people do in their everyday lives.) The vignette technique is better than just asking 'what is your policy about . . .?', because it directs people's attention to the needs of the case and therefore stands some chance of avoiding some of the general rhetoric surrounding the topic. It gives practitioners an anchor for their deliberations, so that they can try to make realistic estimates of what they would say and do in the real case. The use of the postal questionnaire also gives the technique the strength of this kind of survey research, of being able to reach a large number of people in a relatively short space of time and with relatively low use of resources. However, when all is said and done, the fictional case is *not* a real case, and we cannot be *certain* that the outcome in the real case would be the same. The fictional case does not put the respondent under the same kind of pressure as the real one, because the outcome of decisions taken in the fictional case does not have any real costs, and also the information available to the decision-maker is severely limited. This last problem can be overcome by increasing the realism of the situation; Wasoff (1992), for example, investigated lawyers' advice in marital cases by setting up a 'stooge client' with the lawyers' consent – one of the researchers acted the role of the client, instead of details being provided in written form, and so the situation was very close to that of a real consultation. However, this is resource-intensive and loses the survey's advantage of reaching substantial numbers of respondents cheaply.

A further question, for evaluation, is the question of representation (**sampling**). A real attempt was made to get representative samples of users and patients from the three GP practices and to get responses from *all* the district nursing and home help teams which served them – and from all the organizers and team leaders in the whole county, for one of the questionnaires. We do not know how representative the achieved samples were, however, because the report does not tell us much about non-compliance – about the people who refused to fill in questionnaires or be interviewed. It is always a problem that if people who refuse to answer are very different in some respect from those who did comply with the research, then the **descriptive statistics** may be in error in some respects. (In fact there were no refusals; all the patients/clients on the three GPs' lists who were receiving services agreed to be interviewed, and all the home helps and district nursing team members in these three areas cooperated in the research.) Even if the samples were representative of the GP practices, we still have to ask how representative they were of the county as a whole and of the country as a whole. We have no reason to suppose that they are *un*typical, except that the rurality of the location puts service provision under greater stress than in central urban areas, and the researchers did their best to ensure typicality. However, some caution still needs to be exercised in interpreting the figures.

Summary: points for evaluation

1 In any piece of survey research one important question is how well the things which are being counted have been defined – how good the measurement is. There are four sub-questions which might follow from this:

(a) Looking logically at the argument of the paper, have the right things been measured? (Are the concepts correctly **operationalized**?)

(b) Are the factual questions clear and unambiguous, and how likely is it that the respondents have answered them accurately?

(c) Where what is being asked is being taken as a measure or indicator of something underlying, is it a valid indicator? In other words, what is the proof that it does measure what it is claimed to measure? Questions of the artificiality of 'stimulus situations' may validly be asked here.

(d) Looking at the interview or recording session as a social situation of which respondents have to make sense, how likely is it that the sense they make of the task will lead to them giving the information which the argument of the paper needs (as opposed, for instance, to something which is specific to the interview situation and is not likely to have any bearing on any other part of their lives)?

2 How typical is the sample of the population to which the results are to be generalized?

   (a) Was the sampling carried out in such a way that it is likely to be representative, or by a method which makes bias likely?

   (b) Were certain parts of the population excluded from consideration, either deliberately or accidentally (e.g. by non-response to self-completion questionnaire), and what difference might that make to the conclusions?

Exercise 22

Now re-read the two papers in the light of our comments.

Further reading

Community care for older people

Arber, Sara and Ginn, Jay (1991) *Gender and Later Life: A Sociological Analysis of Resources and Constraints*. London: Sage.

Davies, Bleddyn, Bebbington, A. and Charnely, Helen (1990) *Resources, Needs and Outcomes in Community-Based Care*. Aldershot: Gower.

Garrett, G. (1990) *Older People: Their Support and Care*. Basingstoke: Macmillan.

Jamieson, A. (ed.) (1991) *Home Care for Older People in Europe*. Oxford: Oxford University Press.

Jefferys, M. (ed.) (1989) *Growing Old in the Twentieth Century*. London: Routledge.

Phillipson, C., Bernard, M. and Strang, P. (eds) (1986) *Dependency and Interdependency in Old Age: Theoretical Perspectives and Policy Alternatives*. Beckenham: Croom Helm.

CHAPTER SEVEN

READING SECONDARY SOURCES

Using secondary sources
Research paper: Abbott and Tyler (1995)
Standardization and comparison
Summary: points for evaluation
Further reading

Using secondary sources

Like most methods courses and textbooks, we have talked so far as if all research were a matter of going out and collecting fresh data. In fact, the most commonly practised kind of research involves illustrating or supporting an argument by reference to data which have already been collected by someone else, generally for some other purpose. This is known as the secondary use of data, and we refer to the sources as **secondary sources**. Most commonly when we use the term we mean published numerical data – 'statistics', in the original meaning of the term, meaning numerical information about something of interest in the population. Possible sources range widely, from the statistics contained in other people's published research, through various kinds of regular **survey** such as the General Household Survey or the **Census**, and statistics collected for governmental research reasons (e.g. the incidence of certain kinds of infectious diseases), to statistics which are purely a by-product of the administrative process (criminal convictions, admissions to hospital, birth and death statistics, etc.). These are very good sources of information in that they can usually offer a degree of coverage which is beyond the resources of the individual researcher or research team. It would not be possible for you, for example, to count every baby born in the country each year, but the government counts them routinely. The use of secondary sources presents special problems, however, precisely because it is a secondary use; we are often trying to use statistics for purposes for which they were not originally intended. We have to be especially careful, therefore, that the ones we use are **reliable** (i.e. an accurate count of what we want to count, collected in a consistent way), and **valid** for the purposes for which we want to use them.

As a case of unreliable statistics, we might briefly consider the statistics on suicide available from the government publication *Statistics of Deaths Reported to Coroners*. This gives a count of the number of cases where a coroner has determined (with or without the aid of a jury) that the cause of an unexplained death shall be recorded as suicide; that is *precisely* what they count – not the 'real' incidence of suicide, whatever that may mean.

1 Not all suicide cases, almost certainly, are reported to coroners in the first place. If the deceased was under the care of a doctor and the doctor certi- fies the death as being from natural causes, and no other person reports the death as suspicious to the coroner or to the Registrar of Deaths, then the case will never come to the attention of a coroner at all and, there- fore, cannot appear in the statistics.

2 The coroner (and probably the police) will investigate cases of suspicious death before the inquest, and they may find sufficient evidence to justify a suicide verdict.

3 When all the evidence is in, the decision as to whether the case is a sui- cide, an accident or some form of homicide is a subjective one on the part of the coroner (or the jury, if one has been called), and therefore liable to be affected by the personal values of those taking it. This invalidates any sort of class or gender comparison even within one country, because it is all too likely that suicide will seem a more plausible explanation for one class than another, or one gender than another, on a systematic, cultur- ally determined basis. It certainly invalidates comparisons between countries given, for example, the different social consequences of sui- cide in Catholic and Protestant countries.

4 At a more fundamental level, it is not possible even in principle to have an accurate count of suicides. We cannot ask the suicide whether he or she really meant to die. If we give any credence whatsoever to the con- cept of suicide attempts as cries for help, and allow that some attempts which if they had failed would be seen as 'not serious attempts' might accidentally succeed in killing the person concerned, then we cannot ever know whether the person in question died by deliberate self- slaughter.

5 Even if it had been possible to ask, or if an explanatory note has been left, we still cannot be quite sure, because one cannot be quite sure (given any idea of unconscious motivation) that even the victims themselves are in a position fully to explain their actions.

By contrast, the Census is a reliable source of information about the population. There are still some areas in which it may fall down. When counting households, for instance, it relies on its enumerators (data col- lectors) to apply a definition of 'household' consistently, and despite sub- sequent checking we can never be quite certain that this has been done in the case of non-standard households. The count of the homeless is frankly suspect, being carried out by police officers going round the likely haunts of those who sleep rough and trying to get what information they can. In the last instance, moreover, the accuracy of what is put on the form depends on the honesty and understanding of the individual informants. By and large, however, we would be prepared to accept the Census as one of the most reliable of data sources.

The paper which we shall be considering in this chapter is an illustration of what can be done from census data. It uses just two tables from the 1991 Census to explore some quite complicated questions about the employ- ment of women, and particularly of women from 'minority ethnic groups'.

The aim is to test whether the effects of gender and 'race' are additive – two separate kinds of discrimination, with Black women suffering both of them – or whether they **interact** to produce something which is more or less than the expected effect of adding the two together. The answer which emerges from the figures is 'It's more complicated than that!' and the analysis illustrates both the strengths of quantitative work and the amount of knowledge and imagination which is often needed if the results are to be interpreted correctly.

Research paper: Abbott and Tyler (1995)

Exercise 23

You might now read Abbott and Tyler (1995) 'Ethnic variation in the female labour force' (*British Journal of Sociology*, 46: 339–53, or reprinted in Abbott and Sapsford (eds) (1997) *Research into Practice: A Reader for Nurses and the Caring Professions*, 2nd edition). You should not get too deeply involved in the figures when reading the paper – read it for the main conclusions and look to see how the tables support them.

The article starts from premises well established by other research – that gender and 'race' are important factors contributing to the structure of the labour market and sources of discrimination and exploitation within it. 'Ethnic' disadvantage in the labour market is a well established feature, with Black people discriminated against for jobs and likely to finish up, for a given level of qualification, in a lower and worse-paid occupation than a comparable White person. The effect of gender is also well documented. Women are segregated both vertically in the labour market – to some extent excluded from 'higher' (managerial, professional) occupations and from the label of 'skilled' when they are in manual work – and horizontally in terms of there being distinctive 'female' sectors of the market. Women are secretaries, nurses, 'carers', teachers (particularly in primary schools), social workers, shop workers, personal service workers; but they are relatively rarely engineers, scientists, lawyers, accountants, police, army, drivers, miners, skilled factory workers. Or they are semi- or unskilled manual workers in certain trades but not others. While men are clustered in the managerial, administrative and professional grades or in skilled manual work, women are clustered in routine manual work (secretarial and clerical) – which accounts for some 40 per cent of female employment – and in the service sector. Within any given band of employment, women tend to be located at the bottom and men in the higher reaches. More men are self-employed professionals and more women professionals work for a salary. Men are disproportionately represented as head teachers, senior social workers, professors and managers, even in the 'female' employment sectors – the most obvious case being nursing, where few men are nurses but disproportionately many are senior nurses.

The authors' interest was to examine the way in which these two discriminations – by gender and by ethnic group – interact to shape and constrain the location of Black women in the labour market. Such research had been well-nigh impossible in the past, because the target group form such a small proportion of the UK population; in 1991, according to Census data, only 1.5 per cent of the population were Black (of African or Caribbean origin), 1.8 per cent were of Asian origin, 0.2 per cent of Chinese origin, and 0.3 per cent 'others' – a total of less than four per cent of the population, and clearly a much smaller proportion if you count only the women. Thus sample surveys were not able to look at the position of women from minority ethnic groups with any degree of accuracy or perceptiveness, because of the very small numbers involved. However, the 1991 Census asked a question about ethnic origin which was fairly well answered, so Census figures give us information about the whole population in terms of ethnic origin. This paper used the tables of ethic origin by work status and category.

The headline results were that Black women of Caribbean or African origin were more likely to be economically active than White women – more likely, that is, to be in work or to describe themselves as seeking work – and if employed they were more likely to be in full-time jobs than White women. All non-White economically active women, however, were more likely than White women to be currently unemployed or taking a government training scheme offered as a substitute for employment.

We immediately become aware, in looking at these figures, that statistics do not just 'present the facts' but have to be interpreted through a knowledge of how they are collected. The Census counts people as economically active if they say they are currently seeking work or currently have a job. (We may note, incidentally, that there may be cultural differences in whether a married woman describes herself as 'seeking work' when unemployed, so that there can be more than one explanation for some of the observed difference between Black and White women.) Other surveys might count people as unemployed *whether or not* they were seeking work – counting simply the fact of not having a job, rather than trying to count just those who are available for work – and come up with a larger figure for unemployment. On the other hand, another major source of statistics is the count of those *claiming benefit* and *registered* as seeking work, produced by the relevant administrative departments of the government. This gives a smaller figure than the Census, because it excludes those who are seeking work (or would take it if offered it) but have not registered themselves at the relevant office – many of whom may be married women. Which figure you use when assessing unemployment will depend on the purpose for which you are making the assessment, but it is clearly important to think about the source of the figures and what is included in or excluded from a particular source.

A major finding of the analysis presented by Abbott and Tyler is that 'ethnic group' is not a simple, monolithic category when it comes to looking at labour market position. In particular, women from minority ethnic groups are *not* uniformly in the 'lower' employment grades. Women of Pakistani or Chinese origin are overrepresented in managerial and professional grades, compared with women from other ethnic minority groups or with White women, and there are more Chinese women acting as managers or owners of small businesses than there are Chinese men! Thus the interactions between gender and 'race' are clearly not simple ones, and we cannot predict a person's labour market position by simply 'adding the effects together'.

This paper illustrates the major strength of research using published statistics. Using the Census meant that the authors had access to figures they could not possibly have collected for themselves, and a complex research question could be answered by two people, in a fairly short space of time, mostly from just two tables of data. It also illustrates the weakness of such research, however – that you have to work with what is provided, rather than what you might have collected for yourself. What we have is counts of the ethnic group into which respondents are prepared to assign themselves, and their answers to questions about whether they are currently in employment, on a government training scheme, seeking work or, in various ways, not economically active (retired, permanently sick or disabled, a student, a 'full-time housewife', etc.). Using these figures we find that women from some ethnic backgrounds are more likely than White women to be economically active (but less likely to be actually in employment) and more likely to be working full-time, and that women from others are disproportionately to be found in 'higher' employment categories. From this we could be tempted to argue that some groups do not experience discrimination. However, this takes no account of the position of those groups where the women are *not* as likely to be in employment as men, nor of the women's educational and professional qualifications and whether their current occupations are commensurate with them (areas which could have been explored if the authors had been carrying out their own survey). Further, it accepts the grading system of occupations used by the Registrar General and in the Census and is not able to explore precisely *what* jobs White or minority women carried out within a category. Knowing as we do that the Registrar General's schema puts 'air hostess' and 'cafe waitress' in the same category and consigns a one-person computer engineering concern to the same category as a jobbing gardener who works alone, we must at least *wonder* whether some of the attributions to the higher categories conceal discrimination or disadvantage in terms of the precise *kind* of job carried out. Further, we do not know the precise ways in which patriarchal control is exercised over women in different minority ethnic groups, as influenced by cultural heritage, current experience and current structural position. As the authors say,

> it should be noted that this type of analysis does not permit control for factors such as the relationship between educational qualifications and occupational category, or indeed the 'unpicking' of precise occupational position within the broad occupational categories of the Census, so that significant forms of discrimination must necessarily be invisible to it.
>
> (Abbott and Sapsford 1997: 159)

One thing the paper does do, covertly and implicitly, is to question an **ideological** 'taken-for-granted' of research and social practice. 'Black', or 'ethnic minority', are in many ways not descriptive categories but ideological objects – very different people are classed together in the one group, for political reasons rather than because they necessarily have much in common. (It is worth thinking, in this context, about the different uses of 'Black' in French research – where it may often mean someone of Algerian or other North African origin – and in German research, where it may often mean a Turk.) The paper demonstrates just how little the women of different ethnic groups have in common in terms of their labour market position. However, at another level the paper also perpetuates the ideological category. To select people of African, Caribbean, Chinese and other Asian origin as the 'minority ethnic groups' to be considered, and leave out people of Polish, Irish or North American origin, is in itself to perpetuate the notion that these people form a bounded group somehow different from White people of European or North American (but non-British) origin.

Exercise 24

Now re-read the paper in the light of our comments.

Standardization and comparison

One concept which you need when tackling any kind of quantitative research report is that of 'comparing like with like' by **standardizing** the figures – which sounds difficult and abstract but is actually often a very simple process indeed. If you have two sets of figures which are in some way unlike each other, you standardize when you do some simple (or sometimes not so simple!) arithmetic on them to make them easier to compare with each other. The simplest form of standardization is the familiar operation of expressing figures as percentages. If for example you were given the figures on the left of Table 7.1, which group of boys would you say was the greediest? Those in the first column ate more cakes, but there were also more of them. By percentaging, we eliminate (control for) the difference in number of boys, so that we can see clearly that it is Group B which ate proportionately more of their cakes – the figures on the right of the table. Then, in the final line of the table, another form of standardization is demonstrated – reducing the figures to a common base of cakes per boy, again showing that Group B were the greedier. Putting it another way, Group B's boys ate more cakes each, on average, than we would expect if we took Group A as typical.

More complex transformations are necessary when you want to look at underlying causes of a complex phenomenon which are obscured by other, related differences. Take the case of mortality statistics, for example, and the **standardized mortality ratio (SMR)**. The SMR, as its name suggests, is a form of standardization, and it is similar in essence to the notion of cakes per boy in Table 7.1. Eastbourne has a much higher death rate than the country as a whole – per thousand of population, more people die there in

Table 7.1   Two illustrations of standardization
Each boy in two groups was given ten cakes and told to save as many as he could,
but to eat if he was very hungry.

	Actual numbers		Percentages	
Group	A	B	A	B
Number of boys in group	5	2		
Number of cakes available	50	20		
Cakes eaten	15	8	30%	40%
Cakes eaten per boy	3	4		

the course of a year than we would expect from looking at the death rate for the population as a whole. On the other hand, it also has a larger than average population of pensionable age, so on the whole you would expect there to be more deaths. It is also well known that women are hardier than men at all stages of the life-cycle – less likely to die by any given age, and more likely to 'make old bones'. So if we wanted to look at how different Eastbourne's medical services are, using death rates as a basis of comparison, it would hardly be fair to Eastbourne just to take crude death rate as our measure. What we do is to say arbitrarily that the SMR for the population as a whole is 100. Then we look at the area we want to analyse (Eastbourne) and see how its population compares with the country as a whole in terms of age and sex. For each age band in each sex we work out a separate *age- and gender-specific death rate* for the population as a whole – what proportion of men aged 30–39 died in the population as a whole, for instance, what proportion of women aged 30–39, and so on. Then we apply these specific death rates to the numbers in the population of Eastbourne to find out how many deaths we would expect if the age and gender structure of Eastbourne were the same as that of the whole population. We can then compare this **expected figure** with the number who actually died, dividing the one by the other and then multiplying by 100. If the result is less than 100, then Eastbourne has fewer deaths than might have been expected. If it is larger than expected, then it has more deaths than might be expected. We can even say how much less or more: an SMR of 80 would mean that Eastbourne had only 80 per cent of the deaths we would expect if it were similar to the rest of the country in terms of age and sex balance; an SMR of 120 would mean it had 20 per cent more deaths than expected. (Eastbourne actually has a relatively low SMR: its hospital and community practitioners have considerable competence in geriatric medicine.) So the calculation of SMR may be difficult, but the basic idea is a simple one: find out if we have more or less deaths than we would expect after *controlling for* the effects of age and sex.

One thing that standardization does is to allow us to say something quite complicated in one or two figures. For example, instead of saying 'Compare "one out of ten" with "17 out of 340"', we can say 'Compare 10 per cent with 5 per cent', which is much easier to understand. Many complex statistics are used for this reason – to allow us to make precise statements about relationships in a simple manner, as in the case of the standardized mortality ratio.

Another statistical tool of this kind is the correlation coefficient (r), which allows us to express a relationship between two variables as a single figure. Two variables are said to be *associated* or **correlated** if there is a relationship between them such that extreme values on one predict extreme values on the other and a middling value on one predicts a middling value on the other. So height and weight are correlated: all things being equal, taller people weigh more. This is called *positive correlation*, with high values on one variable predicting high values on the other. *Negative correlation* occurs where high values on one variable predict low values on another: an example might be fitness and blood pressure – all things being equal, the less fit you are, the higher your blood pressure. *Perfect* correlation (positive or negative) is said to occur when the values of one variable exactly predict the values of the other – distance covered in a given time is perfectly correlated with speed of running (by definition). Perfect correlation is seldom found in social research, however. When we say that height and weight are correlated, we do not mean that all tall people are heavier than all people shorter than them, but that on the whole the heaviest people will be among the tallest.

The *correlation coefficient* is a mathematical way of expressing the degree to which two variables are correlated – tedious to calculate, but quite easy to understand. A coefficient of correlation carries the value of +1.0 if there is perfect positive correlation between the two variables, –1.0 if there is perfect negative correlation, and zero if there is no correlation at all. The values in between express the degree and direction of correlation, so +0.7 is a reasonably high degree of positive correlation, and –0.2 a reasonably low degree of negative correlation. For those who like playing with their calculators, if you square the correlation coefficient (i.e. multiply it by itself) and multiply the answer by 100, you get *percentage of variance explained*. (The variance is the amount the figures differ among each other.) A perfect correlation of 1.0 or –1.0 explains 100 per cent of the variance. A correlation coefficient of zero explains none. The correlation of 0.7 above explains 49 per cent of the variance, and the one of 0.2 only 4 per cent.

Summary: points for evaluation

1 With secondary-source material, as with any other data, it is very important to understand just how the 'facts' have been collected and to be able to assess the reliability of the source – whether it works accurately and consistently in its data collection.

2 With secondary sources even more than other forms of data the question of validity arises – whether the data collected quite correspond to what the researcher wants to use them for.

3 With secondary-sources data as with other survey-based sources, we should note that the argument which is put forward tends to be based on correlational or **quasi-experimental** logic. Arguments of this kind can

be very strongly suggestive, but they do not, strictly, establish **causation** beyond doubt.

4 However, it is quite possible for an argument of this form to be so strongly suggestive that it may be worth altering social policy and spending social resources on the basis of it. We should always ask ourselves what we can do on the basis of findings as well as what we can conclude.

Further reading

Vital statistics and statistics on health

A basic source of statistics on birth, death, disease, marriage, etc. is the *OPCS Monitor* series, of which specific annual issues deal with specific topics:

DH2 Deaths, by cause
DH4 Deaths from accidents and violence
DH5 Infant and perinatal death statistics
MB2 Infectious diseases
FM1 Birth statistics
FM2 Marriage and divorce statistics

Birth and death statistics may also be found in the *Social Trends* and *Population Trends* (or, for Northern Ireland, *Health and Personal Social Services Statistics for Northern Ireland* and the *Annual Report of the Registrar General for Northern Ireland*). Statistics on illness may be found in *Health and Personal Social Services Statistics*. For figures on health inequalities by class and region see Peter Townsend *et al.* (1990) *Inequalities in Health*. Harmondsworth: Penguin. This volume contains both *The Black Report* and *The Health Divide*, government-funded reports on health a decade apart.

DOING RESEARCH

USING SECONDARY SOURCES

Using libraries – review of literature

Most research reports begin with a section (or sections) which outlines the area of research, explains why it is interesting and/or important, and probably summarizes what is known so far and what the research which is reported has to offer which is new or different. Readers need to know what you can take for granted and build on, and why you choose to look at the problem in the way that you do. For the construction of this section of a report you will have to use the resources of libraries. In fact, you would almost certainly want to do so at a much earlier stage of the research. Reading past research reports and descriptive papers, and more theoretical articles and books, is an important part of the process of refining the research problem and forming ideas about how to carry out the research.

From your point of view, libraries come in two kinds – public and academic. The libraries of universities, colleges and schools of nursing are the better stocked from the point of view of carrying out a search through the 'literature', and if you are a registered student you will have automatic rights to use them. If you are not, however, your access will be limited. Most will allow you reading rights – to look at books and journals on the premises – and some will allow you to borrow books. Many will charge for the privilege. You will have to ask the librarian what is allowed in the particular library which is convenient for you. Public libraries are more accessible, and the larger branches will have some of what you need, but you are unlikely to find that they carry a large stock of publications of the kind you are looking for.

In both kinds of library you will find:

- books, generally arranged according to a subject-based cataloguing system;
- journals, newspapers and other periodicals;
- the catalogue, which lists what the library stocks, by author, title and often subject area;
- abstracts (volumes which contain a complete year-by-year list of publications in a certain area, by author and title, with a brief summary of contents, and generally an index classified by subject-matter to help you locate useful works); for example, *Nursing Abstracts* lists and describes a wide range of research on nursing;
- Annual review journals – for example, *Research in Nursing and Health*;
- other bibliographic instruments – e.g. lists of published works such as *British Books in Print*.

There is a national borrowing network based on the British Library, a copyright library that receives copies of everything published in this country, which also acquires quite a range of works published abroad. Books can be borrowed, and photocopies of journal articles obtained, by what is called 'inter-library loan', and you should talk to the librarian if you need this. Be warned, however, that it can often take quite a lot of time to obtain books or articles by this means, and that there may often be a quite substantial fee for the service unless you are a registered student.

The library of the Royal College of Nursing, in London, has a very large collection of relevant publications. People doing research on health and nursing should contact them if their local facilities are meagre or their subject-area is a very specialized one.

In general, the most useful resource of all in a library is the librarians, who are generally very willing to help the student or researcher.

There are four main 'tricks' for homing in on relevant books and articles reasonably quickly:

1 Identify the catalogue reference which most closely fits the subject-matter of your enquiry (asking the librarian's help if necessary) and just look along the shelves at this point to see what the library has. You will be interested in anything which is fairly recent and/or which obviously bears closely on the question which underlies your research.

2 Browse through the last couple of years' issues of relevant journals for ones which are obviously, by their title, relevant to your work, and ones which you have noticed crop up quite often in the reference lists of other papers and books which you have been reading. (Don't neglect the book reviews, nor publishers' advertisements for books about to be published.)

3 Starting from papers which you have read and found useful, look in the reference lists to identify other articles or books which may be relevant. If they are, when you read them, look in their reference lists in turn for other works. Then look through current journals or abstracts (see below) for the most recent work by the same authors.

4 Use the subject index of the major series of abstracts in your field (ask the librarian if you are not sure) to identify further relevant references. This is the most comprehensive stratagem, but the riskiest in the short term, because you may put in a lot of work locating papers or books which turn

out not to be of immediate relevance. It is a relevant way to proceed if you are writing a book or thesis, or if you are stuck for any references whatsoever, but on the whole it is not a good way to start.

Exercise 25: Literature search

If you have access to a reasonably large library, try your hand at an embryonic literature search. Take one of the papers you read in Section 2 which interested you, and try to identify and locate further articles or books which bear on the same topic.

Finding statistics

A part of the 'literature review' of any research paper will generally comprise an attempt to set the object of study in its context – to say how many of the people concerned there are, what proportion of the population they form, and in general how big the problem is. For this we need the figures which are collected by governmental and other bodies, published and made available in libraries: annual reports of government departments, figures routinely presented to Parliament, regular governmental **surveys** of the population or the economy or the institutions for which government is responsible. We may also need such figures to show how **typical** or **representative** our research samples are of the population which they purport to represent. Indeed, as we saw in the last chapter, it is quite possible to conduct an entire research project on such secondary data. Often it will be the case that using already available statistics is the best way of tackling a research problem; the figures generally give a breadth of coverage that would not be available to the individual researcher without the expenditure of very large amounts of money and time.

Very often the figures you need will be in one or other of the regular annual summary publications. *Social Trends* produces annual 'headline' figures from a wide range of statistical sources and gives an overall picture of the state of the nation. Detailed figures on births, marriages, deaths, family formation and so on can be found in the monthly *Population Trends*, and more localized figures are available in *Regional Trends*. These often include articles analysing and commenting on trends. For the audience of this book, the annually published *Health and Personal Social Services Statistics* is also likely to be an important source.

For more detailed work and for statistics which are harder to find, the 'bible' of the secondary-source researcher is the *Guide to Official Statistics* published from time to time by the Central Statistical Office (CSO). This gives an annotated list of virtually all sets of published official statistics, and some statistics published by non-governmental bodies. Consulting the CSO *Guide* is a normal first step in any secondary-source research, unless you already know your sources very well.

Population and vital statistics

The major source of statistics on the population and its demographic characteristics is the **Census**, held every ten years. (We have already looked at this briefly in the last chapter.) The Census asks every household questions about who is present on Census night, who is usually present, their age, marital status, country of birth, employment, means of transport to work, educational qualifications, where they used to live, the details and amenities of their living accommodation, etc. It is the best source for reliable and authoritative information on the population and their housing in a given area. Results are presented on a regional basis and by county, as well as in national terms (for some of the analyses), and statistics of smaller areas are available on request, in tabular form or in a form amenable to computer analysis. (Some of the more complex analyses are carried out not on the full returns, but on a sample of them.) A limited range of statistics are also available for local authority areas, urban areas, political constituencies, and even wards and parishes.

Happening every ten years, the Census is inevitably out of date for large parts of a decade. More recent information (though generally based on samples rather than the whole population) may be obtained from the monthly Office of Population Censuses and Surveys (OPCS) publication *Population Trends*, from *Regional Trends* if geographically more specific information is required, and from the annual *Social Trends* if all that is required is a broad overview. The other main source of descriptive population statistics, also carried out by OPCS, is the *General Household Survey*, a sample survey of a **panel** of households which asks some of the questions covered in the Census, but also more detailed ones on household amenities and income. A report of the survey is published annually.

There is a strict legal requirement for births and deaths to be reported, so these are among the most **reliable** of the published statistics. *Population Trends* gives numbers of births and deaths by age and gender, noting also numbers of stillbirths and of illegitimate births, and broad summary figures are also given in the annual *Social Trends*. More detailed figures are given in various of the *OPCS Monitors*; you should consult the CSO *Guide* for a list of these. Figures are often given as rates per thousand or ten thousand of the population (or of women of child-bearing age, in the case of births), a more useful way of representing them than simple raw numbers. Death rates may be further adjusted to take account of the age and sex structure of the population under examination – the **standardized mortality ratio**, discussed in the previous chapter, is set at 100 if the group or region's adjusted death rate is identical to the national average. Some statistics for Scotland and Northern Ireland will be found in *Population Trends*, but the major sources here are the *Annual Report of the Registrar General, Scotland* and the *Annual Report of the Registrar General (Northern Ireland)*.

Health and the National Health Service

There are no systematic statistics on the health or disease of the population, but only records of particular illnesses or causes of death. A variety of death figures are available – childhood deaths at various stages around and before birth, causes of death as recorded on death certificates, deaths from accident or violence, occupational mortality, etc. These are reported in *OPCS Monitors* and in a variety of other publications (see the list at the end of the previous chapter, and the CSO *Guide* for more detailed and up-to-date information). Certain infectious diseases have to be reported, and figures for these are given in *Health and Personal Social Services Statistics for England* (or comparable publications for the other countries of Great Britain – see the CSO *Guide*), as are reported cases of sexually transmitted diseases, registered cases of cancer and notifications of congenital malformation. This source also gives numbers of reported pregnancies and numbers of abortions carried out. The *General Household Survey* asks questions on smoking in even-numbered years and publishes the results, and the 1980 and 1982 volumes include data on drinking (which is also covered in summary form in *Social Trends*). Again there are more detailed sources of information which offer a range of analyses, and you should consult the CSO *Guide* for a list of them.

Statistics on the working of the health service are somewhat more comprehensive. Numbers of personnel in the hospital, family practitioner committee and community health branches of the service, and local authority social service, are given in *Health and Personal Social Services Statistics*, as are costs, sources of finance and charges to patients or clients, and a breakdown of hospital beds by location and department. This volume also gives figures on use of hospital treatments, and the age and gender of patients, numbers of general practitioners, the number and cost of prescriptions dispensed, numbers of dentists and incidence of dental treatment, numbers of ophthalmic practitioners and the use (and cost) of their services, the numbers and usage in the ambulance service, and numbers in the school health service and the number of pupils inspected. There are cognate publications for Scotland, Wales and Northern Ireland, and many more specialized sources dealing with particular aspects of the service – again, see the CSO *Guide*.

Social services statistics

The major source here is *Health and Personal Social Services Statistics for England* (and comparable sources for the other countries of the British Isles – see the CSO *Guide*). This gives details of personnel and all the services which have been provided – domiciliary services, residential services, children and young persons in local authority care, housing and homelessness, etc. It also gives numbers of adoptions of children. *Local Government Financial Statistics* gives financial data on the personal social services. Again there are more detailed sources, for which you should consult the CSO *Guide*.

> **Exercise 26: Exploring secondary data**
>
> If you have an adequate library available, why not spend a few hours seeing what you can get out of available statistics. Pick some limited area of enquiry, look for relevant figures in the overall summary volumes such as *Social Trends*, look in the CSO *Guide* to see what else might be available and follow it up.

Problems with published statistics

Published statistics are a very strong source of information – the only available one for making comparisons over extended periods of time, unless you have a very long time in which to conduct your research, and with a 'sample size' that you are very unlikely to be able to match. There are problems, however, connected with the ways in which they are assembled and the purposes for which they are collected, which mean they have to be treated with even more caution than other sources of information.

The first problem is the question of **reliability**: are the statistics collected in a consistent way, so that one year's figures are comparable with another's? There may be several stages in a statistic's 'history' at which an individual's discretion comes into play, and this could be exercised in different ways from year to year, from place to place and from person to person. There are also gross changes of law, practice and the state of knowledge to contend with. Diagnosis of disease or handicap, for example, depends on someone presenting himself or herself to a doctor, who then exercises medical judgement as to whether a diagnosable condition is present and, if so, what it is. There are advances of medical knowledge which will change particular diagnostic practice from time to time. Reliability may also be influenced by more social factors. For example, now that there are incentives to doctors for screening of women for cervical cancer, cases will be diagnosed earlier and there will be a temporary rise in the statistics – fewer cases will wait for the diagnosis until the condition becomes acute. The government statistics on numbers of deaths are reliable, being taken from counts of death certificates. The statistics on cause of death are also taken from death certificates, however, and these are not reliable: they depend on the potentially fallible diagnosis of doctors, plus an additional level of 'clerical discretion', where more than one cause is recorded and a clerk will have to decide which to take as the primary one. All survey questions – even apparently simple ones such as 'How would you describe your ethnic origin?' Or 'Have you ever been raped?' – have to be scrutinized to see whether fashions in avowal or differential pay-offs for answering one way or the other might change the pattern of answers over time, even if the underlying 'facts' had not changed. Information collected by some government department, often for quite different purposes, needs to be scrutinized even more carefully.

This leads into the question of **validity** – do the statistics measure what they purport to measure? Putting it another way, is what they measure what you want to consider in your research? Diagnostic statistics, for example, measure not the extent of a given disease, but the extent to which it has been diagnosed, and diagnosis is not an automatic process, but one involving human decision-making. The statistics are very likely to be correlated with the real extent of disease – to go up when it goes up and down when it goes down – but the relationship could be quite a loose one, and small changes are as likely as not to be the result of a change in reporting or recording practice. So we need to remember that what we are measuring is, in part, a social construction, not a 'fact', and that there is error in the figures.

Another aspect of the validity question concerns the way that we tend to use what is available, even if it does not quite match up to what we need. In the Abbott and Tyler paper discussed in the last chapter the authors had to use the Census occupational categories simply because they were available. Abbott and Tyler were well aware, however, that these are not well designed for discriminating between women's jobs and tend to 'lump together' occupational positions which are in some ways very different, so that there could be differences between Black and White women which are concealed by their aggregation into the same set of categories. As another example, we might assess the efficiency of hospitals by their throughput of patients and/or the number of patients treated for a given cost, but this would take no account of the quality of treatment. It is very easy to distort the original research question in the interests of using available statistics, or even to miss the core of it altogether.

The moral is that we must always scrutinize the secondary statistics which we are considering with at least as much care as we would scrutinize methods of data collection we intend to use ourselves first-hand. Are the figures likely to be consistently and reliably collected? Do they measure what they purport to measure? Do they measure what *we* want to measure? Will the use of them in any way distort or prejudice the analysis of the original question? If so, what other figures can we use to overcome this, or what research ought we to go on and do to supplement what we can learn from the figures?

'Qualitative' sources

We have talked so far as if all secondary analysis is carried out on published statistics. It is also possible, however, to do qualitative secondary analysis, looking at what people have written or what has been written about them. Studying social policy, for example, government reports and White Papers can be a rich source of information, and for more detailed work one can go to *Hansard*, the daily record of what is said in Parliament, or to the newspapers (*The Times* and *The Guardian* have an annual index which makes it relatively easy to track down the date of 'policy events' – or you may be able to access a CD-ROM version, in which case you can use computerized search facilities). Professional journals can also be very useful in this respect. One should remember that what is presented is what the policy-makers say – how they justify what they are doing – and the criticisms that have been made from a range of entrenched positions; such work is seldom to be taken as a purely factual source of information. In this, however, they differ little from any other qualitative source; it is always necessary to remember that people give *accounts* of their lives and actions, not straight factual reports.

With this same qualification, people's own personal accounts can also help to 'flesh out' figures or can be used as a source in their own right: autobiographies, published collections of letters, diaries, even novels can help to give some feel for what a situation or condition is like 'from the inside' in circumstances where interviewing is not possible. One may also go to reports of ethnographic research for summarized accounts of other people's interviewing. Thus the literature review can also be a form of data collection.

Exercise 27: Exploring qualitative sources

Taking the topic which you explored in Exercise 25, spend a few hours in a large library looking for anything qualitative which bears on it – diaries, letters, autobiographies, ethnographic research reports, official pronouncements. (In other words, get started on a literature review.) See what these add to the quantitative material you have developed.

Summary

1 A fair amount of research analysis can be done without carrying out research fieldwork – through examination of the research of others and by analysis of figures collected and published by government and other agencies.

2 When using these figures – particularly those collected as a by-product of administration rather than by specifically designed surveys – care has to be taken to ensure that the figures are reliable over time and as measures of what they purport to measure. To ensure this, a fair amount has to be known about how the figures are collected.

3 Even where figures are reliable measures of what they claim to measure, care must still be taken that they are valid for the *researcher's* purpose.

4 Sources other than figures – diaries, letters, newspaper articles, speeches, even novels – can also cast useful light on research questions.

Further reading

Hakim, Catherine (1987) *Research Design: Strategies and Choices in the Design of Social Research*. London: Routledge (Chapters 2 and 4).

Hindess, Barry (1973) *The Use of Official Statistics in Sociology*. London: Macmillan.

Irvine, John, Miles, Ian and Evans, Jeff (eds) (1979) *Demystifying Social Statistics*. London: Pluto Press.

McLeod, C.J. and Slodatski, A.N. (1978) How to find out: a guide to searching the nursing literature, *Nursing Times*, 74(6): 21–3.

Plummer, Kenneth (1983) *Documents of Life*. London: Allen and Unwin.

Useful journals for reports of nursing research

Nursing Standard
Nursing Times

British Journal of Midwifery
British Journal of Nursing
Health Visiting Journal
Journal of Advanced Nursing
Nurse Education Today
Nurse Researcher
Surgical Nurse

Social Science and Medicine
Social Sciences in Health
Sociology of Health and Illness

See also, for summaries of research studies, *Nursing Abstracts*.

SURVEY RESEARCH: DESIGN AND SAMPLING

In this chapter we have in mind the sort of research that a practitioner might do in his or her own institution:

1 **surveying** the attitudes of the client population to a service;
2 comparing two groups of clients to see, for example, whether the medical and care needs of elderly men are different from those of elderly women, or whether Black families have different social-work needs from White ones (a sort of **case-control study** of social needs);
3 trying to predict outcomes or looking for **causal** links (e.g. whether some forms of nursing care are more effective than others at achieving a desired end, or whether clients who make repeated use of a counselling service differ systematically from those who come once and then drop out).

We shall also look at how respondents are selected, how **observation/ interview schedules** are constructed (including the construction of attitude and personality scales), what problems for the interpretation of the data can usefully be anticipated at the design stage and the eventual use of **questionnaires** in the field.

The usual stages of survey design are:

1 Formulating the 'problem' or area of study as precisely as possible, probably after:
  (a) reviewing the literature;
  (b) a first **pilot** stage of talking to potential respondents in a fairly open

and unstructured way about the topic(s) of the survey, to get their ideas and some notion of the terminology they use;

(c) where the research is to be carried out in a limited number of settings (e.g. one or a few institutions), spending some time there familiarizing yourself with what goes on.

2 Selecting the sample of respondents or settings, or devising rules for how a sample is to be picked.

3 Deciding on the best mode of 'delivery' – whether you are going to observe behaviour in a systematic way or ask questions; and, if you decide on a questionnaire, whether it will be administered by an interviewer or sent by post for self-completion or delivered by some other means. At this time you would plan what to do about refusals and non-response – whether and when to send follow-up letters, for instance, and whether it is possible to collect any descriptive information about people who refuse to cooperate.

4 Thinking carefully about what descriptive ('demographic') information might be necessary or useful – age, gender, social class, etc. – and precisely how to record it.

5 Thinking what alternative explanations might be offered for any results you obtain, and what extra information you need to collect to explore them.

6 Designing the questionnaire or observation schedule. If this includes measurement scales not in common use, a second stage of pilot work would be needed, to check on the *validity* of the measures (looking for evidence that they do measure what you want) and their *reliability* (that they produce fairly stable and consistent results).

7 In a final pilot stage you would try out the questionnaire or schedule, to identify and deal with problems in its administration. You would also, at this stage, think about how the results are to be analysed, to make sure the data will be recorded in a suitable form.

These stages are described with the usual **cross-sectional** survey in mind, wanting to know what is the case at present and asking a sample of people about it in a **one-shot survey** design. When looking, for example, at changes over time, more sophisticated designs may be required, because of problems of memory and how the present tends to reconstruct the past (see Chapter 6). The two classic ways round this kind of problem are:

1 repeated cross-sections – drawing fresh samples at each time-period, and asking about the present, e.g. sampling a population before broadcast television is introduced to an area, sampling it again afterwards, and comparing the two sets of results;

2 **panel** or **cohort** designs – taking a group of people and asking them questions at designated time-periods, e.g. taking a sample before broadcast television is introduced to an area and questioning the same people again afterwards.

(We tend to talk of 'cohort studies' where the sample purports to be representative of an age group, and otherwise of 'panel studies'.) The panel or cohort study is superior in design terms, but more difficult to set up and maintain.

Most of this chapter will be about questionnaires – asking people questions about themselves and what they think and believe. We should start off by pointing out, however, that surveys do not *have* to ask people questions. The systematic observation of behaviour is an equally important survey technique, and where it is applicable it may be a stronger approach than verbal questioning, because you do not have the difficulty of interpreting the sense which respondents have made of the questions and what they meant by their answers. As a survey technique, observation must be systematic – it must entail counting or measuring behaviours in some consistent and **reliable** fashion. If you have to construct a classification system for yourself, your research would be preceded by a period of more general observation, to obtain a list of the behaviours which can be observed and to work out ways of defining them tightly. Often one researcher will devise a coding system and have it tried out by other researchers; if they can also apply it consistently, then the system is a reasonably reliable one and not just the exteriorization of its author's fancies and prejudices. A further period of observation would then follow, in which all those who were destined to use the system practised it, preferably together and on the same 'cases', until a consistent level of performance emerged; this stage of training and practice would be equally necessary even if you were using another researcher's classification system. A better stratagem is to video the behaviour and do the classification afterwards. This lets you work over the same scene several times, with colleagues, until you reach agreement about what is going on.

Selecting respondents

The ideal 'sample survey' is a **census** – questioning every member of a population (every nurse or patient in a hospital, every client on the caseload, every household in an area). This is seldom practical, however, and so researchers have to **sample** their populations. Very many of the surveys of opinion with whose results we are bombarded by newspapers and manufacturers, however, are grounded in quite inadequate samples. **Market researchers**, for example, may ask their questions of people who pass in the city street, generally during the day. Such people are not typical of the population as a whole: they are those who happen to be on the street at the time, and probably underrepresent people in full-time employment, people at schools or colleges, people who shop locally rather than in the city centre, and so on. Alternatively, they sometimes go from house to house in selected streets. This is a better stratagem, provided that all times of the day and days of the week are covered, but if not, then they are again unlikely to draw **representative** samples, because they will exclude those who are not present at the time in question. Newspaper 'surveys' are often based on even less representative 'volunteer' samples – those who bother to answer a request for information, or those who write spontaneously about something that excites or annoys them. There are better ways of working than these – methods more likely to generate samples which are representative of their populations.

Random sampling

The best kind of sample for survey work is the **random** sample – one drawn from a complete list of the population (i.e. of those to whom we want the results to generalize) in such a way that every member of it has an equal chance of being represented and it is chance that determines which particular members are selected. A sample drawn in this way cannot be seen as influenced by the views and expectations of the researcher – you cannot pick a random sample deliberately in such a way as to prove your own views – and, provided it is fairly large, it stands a good chance of resembling the population from which it is drawn. So if you were looking at some characteristics of your clients, a very good way to proceed would be to obtain a complete list of the current population of clients or of people who have come in over the past months or years and, if the population is small, put all the names in a box, shake it well and draw out as many cases as you want for your sample. If the population is larger than that, you might want to take every nth name, from a randomly chosen starting point – for example, every tenth name, if you wanted a sample of 100 from a population of 1000.

Better still is to resort to a table of random numbers. These are published in all sets of statistical tables and most statistics textbooks, and they consist essentially of a string of numbers with no discernible pattern to them – e.g. 31415873920408279 . . . They may be arranged in sets of five or ten, in columns down the page. All you need to know, to pick a sample using them, is the size of your population and the desired size of sample. Say your population was 10,000, and you wanted a sample of 100. If you picked every hundredth case (as 10,000/100 = 100) you would get the right size of sample, but there might be some pattern to which cases came up a hundred apart; and if the population were actually 10,030, the last 30 cases would stand no chance at all of being selected. So you can use the first four numbers in the table to determine a random starting point: if they were 0001, you would start with the first case, but in this case they are 3141, so you start with the 3141st. Now you could take every hundredth case. Cleverer still is to divide up the population into hundreds and take the nth case from each hundred according to the next pair of random numbers – the 58th from the first hundred, the 73rd from the next hundred, and so on. (When you get to the last case on the list, you carry on counting from the beginning again, as if the cases were arranged in a circle.) This kind of procedure gives you absolutely the least chance of picking a sample which is in any way systematically biased.

If there is no complete list of the population, you might be able to draw a sample by taking the next n cases to come in (e.g. the next 50 cases, if you want a sample of 50), provided cases come in randomly and there is no systematic pattern to the order in which they are received. This last point is crucial, however, and you need to think very carefully about the possibility of patterns occurring – to use your researcher's imagination to think what might be happening. If you took the next 50 cases to come in to the casualty department of a hospital, for example, and you picked the period just after a disputed football match, you would get a very different sample from one drawn in the days immediately preceding Christmas (more victims of fights in the former case, and more victims of drunken driving in the latter). Different kinds of cases come in at night than during the day. It would clearly be best, if you want a representative sample, to preselect times of the day, days of the week and weeks of the year, randomly, and use these as your 'collection points'. Wherever there is any possibility of patterns occurring in a population list or a series of admissions, you should make sure that your selection procedures are random enough to overcome it, and there is no single and simple way of doing so.

Because the random sample *is* random, drawn by chance, it is reasonably likely to be roughly representative of the population, but only roughly. It is possible to improve the representation by a process known as **stratification** – separately sampling the strata or layers of the population, using a variable known to be of some importance. If you draw a random sample of a year's hospital admissions, for example, there is every likelihood that your sample will be roughly representative of the population in terms of numbers of males and females, but only roughly. If you know that gender is an important variable in terms of your research question, you can improve the representative nature of your sample in this respect by drawing separate samples of males and females, in numbers proportionate to the numbers of the two in the population.

Cluster sampling

Frequently, when drawing samples from 'the world at large', rather than a particular institution or setting, a random sample is not appropriate because there is no list of the population from which to draw it, or because the geographical spread of a true random sample would be too great for any researcher to handle. A random sample of 500 housewives scattered across the British Isles would not give more than one or two in each town, and a national random sample of schoolchildren or hospital patients would not be much more accessible. Here we often resort to a process called **cluster sampling** – picking geographical clusters, then sampling within them. If you wanted a national sample of hospital patients, for example, you might pick five or ten hospitals at random and then take a sample of patients within the sampled hospitals. If you wanted a sample of the people in a town, you might pick three or four districts at random, and within them three or four streets, and within them three or four houses, and then interview all the people in the designated houses. There is a risk that your sample will be unrepresentative because the range is constricted – if certain sorts of people occur according to some geographical pattern, then you may oversample those sorts of people and undersample others. However, you can apply the principle of stratification to overcome this risk by selecting your clusters according to some sensible system. If you were sampling within a town, for example, you would make sure to pick some inner-urban areas and some suburban ones, and to select a mix of working-class areas and middle-class ones. If you were sampling hospitals, you would make sure that all types of hospital were represented.

Quota sampling

When nothing else is practicable we tend to resort to **quota sampling**. This is a procedure where we seek to obtain a representative sample of the population by setting up 'quotas', by sets of important variables, which match the population. We might set out, for example, to interview so many elderly middle-class women, so many elderly middle-class men, so many middle-aged middle-class women, and so on. This procedure will guarantee that the sample is representative with respect to the variables which are used to form the quotas. However, there is no control over other variables – interviewers may select whom they like to fill the quotas provided that the quota design is adhered to. Quite serious biases can, therefore, creep into the sampling. For example, in an Open University student survey (see Abbott and Sapsford 1987a) the student interviewers were set a quota design by age, social class and gender, and they matched it fairly exactly. However, the respondents whom they interviewed turned out overall to be better educated than the average, there were substantially more women in full-time employment than one would expect, and women in routine non-manual work were somewhat underrepresented. This pattern undoubtedly reflects the kinds of people Open University students find easy to locate and interview.

There are a number of ways in which quota sampling can be improved, if the interviewer is prepared to expend the effort. For example, an additional element of stratification may be introduced into samples of households by sampling from a variety of areas rather than allowing the quota to be filled from a single area. Time-periods can be randomized or systematically sampled, to minimize the risk of missing certain kinds of people because of their hours of work. A random element can be introduced – picking streets or postcodes at random as starting points. Nevertheless, and with all these improvements, quota sampling remains inherently inferior to random sampling as a way of guaranteeing a sample representative of its population.

It remains a widely used procedure in market research, however, because of its comparative ease and cheapness: there is no need for a complete list of the population to act as a sampling frame, and interviewers do not need to call back if they find a given respondent not at home but can replace him or her with someone else of the right characteristics. In political opinion research, quota sampling has almost entirely replaced more random methods because it has been found that the improvement of prediction given by the latter is too slight in this area of research to justify the extra cost (see McKee 1981).

Exercise 28: Sampling

The first six pages of the 'residential' section of your telephone directory will be the population for this exercise (or some other list with at least 200 names and addresses on it). Count the number of names overall, and also (a) how many of the names have the letter 'a' as the second or third letter of the main surname of the entry, and (b) how many of the addresses list a house *name* of some sort instead of a house *number*. Then take two types of sample:

1 do the same counts for the first 50 names in the list;
2 do the same counts for a random sample of 50 drawn using a table of random numbers.

Compare the results. Which type of sample comes closest to matching the population?

Devising the questions

If you are asking questions rather than observing behaviour, you need a questionnaire. (This holds even if you are interrogating not people, but files or documents; you still need a consistent list of questions to ask about them and a consistent way of recording the answers.) This will contain, broadly, three sorts of questions:

1 There will be demographic questions – age, gender, occupational details (for coding social class), and other explanatory or descriptive variables about people's lives that you are going to need at the analysis stage, such as where they live, the level of their education, etc. You will probably *pre-code* these – work out the possible range of answers and set up categories with the question, so that all that has to be done is to ring a number or tick a box. Be careful, however, to ensure:
   (a) that all possible answers are covered (you may need categories for 'don't know' and/or 'refused to answer');
   (b) that categories do not overlap (age is coded, e.g. as 20–29, 30–39, etc., not 20–30, 30–40, etc., because in the latter coding scheme the code for someone aged 30 is ambiguous); and
   (c) that you will get a reasonably even distribution of responses between the categories of a variable.
   If you do not know the age distribution of your population in advance, for example, it is better to record the actual age in years (or even years and months, for children) and work out categories afterwards.
2 There will be factual questions about people's past histories: whether they have been burgled in the past, when and for what they have been in hospital, their work histories, or whatever. The two problems here, both aspects of validity of measurement, are (a) definition and (b) memory. It is of paramount importance that you define precisely what you mean by the event or happening on which your respondents are to report; other-wise, differences between groups may be due to differences of interpreta-tion, not differences of experience. Secondly, memory for the past is unreliable; people usually remember what has happened to them, but often not precisely when. So it is unwise to ask how many times x has happened 'in the last year'; precisely anchored time-periods such as 'since Christmas' are to be preferred.

3 Questions about attitudes and beliefs – these are more complex than they may at first appear, and there are several ways of proceeding. We shall talk about them in the next section.

Measuring attitudes

Much survey research is concerned with the measurement of attitudes, beliefs, opinions, intentions, etc. If you think of attitudes as something a person has and can report on, then the best way of getting at them is quite simply to ask about them. Much market research takes this stance: 'Which of these two coffees do you prefer?', 'Which would you buy, if they were the same price?' Much political research does likewise: 'How would you vote if there were a general election tomorrow?' The Cornish survey which we examined in Section 2 asked straightforwardly for people's opinions about service provision, as well as about their factual experiences. The only technical problem, in this approach, is to phrase the questions clearly, unambiguously and in such a way that the answers can readily be understood by the researcher.

Another view of the area of attitudes/beliefs/intentions would be to regard an attitude as something that a person has, but is not necessarily able to report – a complex of beliefs and tendencies to behave in certain ways, bound together from an outsider's point of view, but not necessarily apparent to the insider's conscious thought-processes. In that case you would want to find or construct some sort of 'measuring instrument'. You would administer a list of questions which can be shown to be 'symptomatic' of the attitude in question in a number of people, and add the answers together in some way to give a score. Many clinical scales are of this kind: they seek to measure a mental state (e.g. depression) by asking a number of relatively innocuous questions which people who have that particular state typically answer in one way – e.g. 'Do you often feel unhappy?', 'Do you often cry for no reason?', 'Do you have difficulty in sleeping?' You might want to adopt this tactic if the question which underlies your scale is a sensitive one which might offend the respondent, or if there are very strong social norms prompting the respondent to answer in a particular direction.

One way of constructing such a scale is to get a panel of experts in the area to generate a pool of statements which they would see as symptomatic of the attitude or mental state, and use the ones on which the experts appeared to agree. A second and more common way of proceeding is to generate a large pool of items which have 'face validity' – they look at least as if they ought to measure what is required. You then go through at least four stages of pilot work.

1 You administer the items to a group of people (about 20?), getting them to score them on a seven-point scale from, for example, 'very true of me' to 'not at all true of me'. You throw out all those items which tend to attract scores in the middle of the scale from everyone, because they will not help to discriminate any group from any other.

2 You administer the remaining items to two separate groups who can be guaranteed to differ from each other on the variable which the scale is measuring – for example, if you were measuring 'satisfaction with the service we provide' you might pick ten people who have taken the trouble to come and tell you afterwards how good the service was and the ten people who had complained most virulently. You would keep the items which are consistently, on average, answered one way by one group and the other by the other, throwing out those items which did not discriminate.

3 You would retest your original group, a little time afterwards, to see if they gave similar answers (a test of reliability).

4 You would validate the final scale by finding two more groups who undoubtedly differed on the variable in question and seeing if the scale differentiated between them (to ensure that you are not just capitalizing on a chance set of differences in the first pair of groups).

If you had professional resources at your disposal there are two more things you might well do:

5 You might get scores from a large sample of the normal population and from large samples of people who would be expected to score particularly high or low, to establish the normal range of scores and what might be expected of extreme groups.

6 Taking this fairly large data-set, you might subject it to *factor analysis*, a statistical procedure which tests whether all the items **correlate** together (the extent to which they are measuring the same thing) or whether one can distinguish groups of items which correlate with others within the group, but less so with items outside the group (in which case your scale may be measuring more than one variable).

The final scale is demonstrably **valid** and **reliable**. To the extent that these stages have not been undertaken, this cannot be asserted.

Yet another way of looking at attitudes, beliefs and intentions is to see them as products of how the respondent sees the world – what sort of a world he or she thinks we live in, with reference to your area of interest. One can get at people's ways of classifying their world, their 'constructs', by a technique devised by the American psychologist George Kelly (e.g. 1955), known as the Role Repertory Grid. This was originally devised for thera-peutic interviews, but has since been widely used for a range of psycho-logical studies of people and how they see the world, and even in market research (to explore 'brand images'). For an introduction to Kelly's theories and to uses of the Grid, see Bannister and Fransella (1980). A related tech-nique is the semantic differential scale pioneered by Osgood *et al.* (1967), where sets of *supplied* adjectives form the scales on which people, groups or objects of interest are to be rated. The adjectives typically include some of very general reference (e.g. warm/cold, strong/weak) and perhaps some more specific to the particular research topic.

Finally, a useful way of getting at difficult concepts unobtrusively is by the use of what are known as 'projective techniques' – segments of 'verbal behaviour' into which respondents may be seen as projecting or expressing some aspect of mentality. One classic, for example, is the TAT (Thematic

Apperception Test), which consists of a series of ambiguous pictures looking something like magazine illustrations. The respondent is asked to write or narrate the story illustrated by each picture, and it is argued that what appears in the story (not being supplied by the pictures, which are as near neutral in content as possible) expresses something about the respondent. For example, a picture of two men in a room might be seen as brothers at home, or as two colleagues conspiring, or as a homosexual affair, or two people planning to start a successful small business, or . . . The original use of this test was to measure 'achievement motivation' by the amount of achievement-oriented imagery that was produced (McClelland *et al.* 1953). Another example would be the use of photographs to measure affective flattening – getting people to describe what they saw in pairs of photographs of people and seeing the extent to which they did or did not impute emotions to the subjects of them (Dixon 1967; Sapsford 1983).

Anticipating problems

Non-response

Nearly all surveys have a problem of non-response: people refuse to answer, or randomly chosen respondents cannot be contacted, or if you left questionnaires to be filled in by the respondents some of them will not bother to do so. It would be very destructive of a survey's claims to represent the views of a population if the non-response rate were very large, and particularly if the non-respondents were not a random subset of the sample – if particular kinds of people tended not to respond. There is a certain amount you can do about this problem at the fieldwork stage and we shall discuss this later. Two precautions can be taken at the design stage, however. First, it may be possible to anticipate which kinds of people may not respond and to oversample them: in a questionnaire about the banning of smoking at work, for example, you might deliberately set out to question more smokers than would be needed to represent their proportion of the population, anticipating that many smokers will be hostile to the purpose of the questionnaire. (This assumes, of course, that you know the population distribution and that you can reliably identify smokers and non-smokers beforehand.) This kind of *disproportionate stratification* is also useful for making sure that rare groups in the population are adequately represented. The second tactic is to try to find out at least basic demographic characteristics even of the non-responders, so that you can compare them with the respondents and see if they differ in any significant way. If you are interviewing face to face it should be possible to note gender and estimate age and even rough social class. If you are sending out questionnaires and ensuring confidentiality by *not* asking for names and addresses to be sent in, you might still get the postcode or area of town on the respondents' questionnaires, and if you kept a note of how many you dispatched to each postcode or area of town then you can at least see if there is any geographical inequality in the response. (A directory of postcodes is kept in every central post office.)

Reactivity

A second problem which must be anticipated at the design stage is **reactivity**, the risk that some of the answers will be prompted by the way the questionnaire is designed or delivered. You will take great pains at the design stage, for example, to avoid social desirability effects – the tendency of people to 'be in favour of honour and virtue' and to give answers that will represent them as respectable and socially conforming in the eyes of the researcher – by finding ways of phrasing questions which allow the socially less unacceptable responses to seem acceptable. You will avoid too many questions which could naturally be answered 'yes' or 'no'. You would be very sure not to suggest in your question-wording what answer you expect the informant to give. You would also be careful of the order of questions, so that the answer to one question is not suggested by the answer to a previous one.

Alternative explanations

Finally, you need to collect a certain number of demographic variables to test for whether they provide alternative explanations for your results to the explanation which you propose to put forward. If you were examining the relationship between unemployment and certain kinds of 'health behaviour', for example, it might be that poverty provided a more comprehensive explanation than unemployment – that all people in poverty showed the behaviour in question, whether or not they were registered as unemployed. You would, therefore, need to collect some kind of measure of household income, to check whether this was the case. You would also want to collect the obvious demographic characteristics – age, gender, social class, etc. – in order to be able to check that your sample is typical of the population.

Exercise 29: Questionnaire design

Try your hand at designing a questionnaire. Imagine you are commissioned to examine clients'/patients'/customers' satisfaction with the service your agency or firm provides (if you work for an agency or firm), or with a service which you or your family receive (e.g. the service provided by your local primary school). Think carefully what this 'service' is – how many different things the agency or firm does, and the different goals which the clients, etc. might have. (You may need to talk to some people before you start.) Think also who the clients actually are – in the case of a school, for example, are the clients children, or parents, or the education authority, or all of these? Then work out what questions you need to ask, including demographic variables for describing the population, checking on the quality of the sampling and looking for patterns in the results. (You may need different questionnaires for the different kinds of 'client', if their interests are

different.) Think carefully how you would ask the questions, for
maximum acceptability to the respondents and maximum clarity when
you come to analyse the results. If you are able, try your draft out on
three or four appropriate people, and see what changes you want to
make to it after you have seen their responses.

Doing the research

An essential element of research design which we have not yet discussed
(because it affects fieldwork even more than design) is the notional
'research contract' between you and your respondents. You will, of course,
have ensured that your research procedures will not cause pain or distress
to informants, but what are you going to tell them about the research? Are
you asking questions to collect data, regarding what you do with the data
as in a sense none of their business? Or are you adopting a fully collaborative stance, taking them fully into your confidence, carrying out the work
as much to further their interests as your own and regarding the work as in
some sense joint property? If the latter, have you worked out what form the
collaboration will take? Will they be collaborating in the writing of the
report? Will they have free access to each other's data (see 'confidentiality',
below)? If they disagree with your interpretation of the data, do they have
the right to change what is reported, or to have their disagreement registered, or are their comments to be only advisory? If you enter into a collaboration, the rules must be clear to all parties.

It is general practice to promise respondents *confidentiality* – that only
you will be able to match up names and questionnaires, and that the
information will never be used in such a way that the respondent can be
identified. You will need to think carefully about building in procedures
which ensure that this is the case – for example, sampling widely enough
that no individual is unique. Confidentiality is particularly important if
the respondents stand to lose by being identified – if, for example, they are
patients or clients of your agency, or working colleagues, and their views
could be held against them by 'management'. (Sometimes respondents
will not *want* confidentiality – when they want their specific complaints to
be dealt with, for example.)

Also a design matter, as well as an aspect of fieldwork, is precisely how
you intend to deliver the questionnaire. Will you take it round to respondents yourself and ask them the questions, filling in the answers yourself?
Will you use other (perhaps paid) people as interviewers? Will you hand it
out personally, but ask them to fill it in for themselves and return it to you?
Or will you post it to them and ask them to return it? Each of these methods
has advantages as well as disadvantages. If you are your own interviewer,
you can have maximal confidence in the data. You will also probably get a
fairly low refusal rate. On the other hand, you cannot cover very many
cases. Postal delivery is the best method for reaching a wide target population, but the refusal/non-response rate is generally very high; 50 per cent

response would be considered quite high for a postal survey. You will, therefore, do everything you can to increase response rate if you adopt the postal strategy: including a stamped addressed envelope for the return of the form, and writing again, perhaps two or three times, to people who do not respond to the first letter. (This is, of course, impossible unless you are sending the questionnaire to preselected named individuals.) Delivering the questionnaire yourself improves the response rate, but there are still problems. Finally, using others as your interviewers can give you the advantages of personal interviewing but allow you to cover more cases than you could manage by yourself. It may, indeed, be the only way to obtain face-to-face interviews if you are not an appropriate person to be carrying out the interviews yourself. For example, it is better to have a Black interviewer when approaching Black people and a young interviewer when approaching young people – respondents are more at their ease and less likely to give an 'official response'. On the other hand, it is very important that the interviewers be trained to use the questionnaire all in the same way; otherwise differences might be due to characteristics of the interviewers' behaviour rather than characteristics of the respondents.

This question of training also applies to you yourself, if you are administering your own questionnaire. The whole point of this approach is that data shall be collected in a uniform manner from all respondents – that they all answered the same questionnaire, administered in the same fashion. (This is another argument against postal delivery – that you cannot control the conditions under which the questionnaire is filled in.) It is quite vital that all who are to administer the questionnaire know exactly what to do with each question, including the extent to which it is legitimate to explain what is meant and the extent to which they may be required to prompt respondents for more information. The questionnaire must be as standardized a measuring instrument as a thermometer, if we are to put complete confidence in its results.

Finally, we cannot overstress the importance of pilot work. All questionnaires should be tried out, to see what could go wrong, before being administered to the sample at large. It is particularly important to pilot questions, scales, etc. which are intended to measure aspects of attitude, intention or personality. These are of little value as evidence if you cannot demonstrate they are reliable (answered the same way by the same informants over a period of time short enough that change would not be expected) and valid as measures of what you claim that they measure.

Summary

1 If a census (survey of 100 per cent of potential respondents) is not feasible, then surveys have to be based on a sample of the population. A *random* sample drawn from a complete list of the population yields results which are most likely to be representative of the population. *Stratification* may be used to improve the precision of the sampling, where a variable is known to be of importance to the research.

2 When true random sampling is not possible, *cluster* sampling – selecting geographical clusters and sampling within them – may be substituted, but at the risk of some loss of the ability to cover the full range of variation in the population. Alternatively, a *quota* sample may be selected to be representative of the population in terms of variables known to be important – but there is a strong risk that it will be unrepresentative in other respects because the selection of cases to fill the quotas is left to the interviewers.

3 However good the sampling, non-response may render the achieved sample unrepresentative of the population. It is essential to take all possible steps to minimize non-response and to try to record at least basic demographic characteristics of those who refuse to cooperate or cannot be located, to the extent that this is possible.

4 Survey questions may vary from very direct and open enquiries – demographic questions about age, gender, etc., or straightforward questions about behaviours or beliefs – to complex scales made up of items known to correlate with some aspect of personality or attitude. Even with the straightforward questions it is necessary to think carefully about how they will be understood by the respondents and what effect they will have on them. A pilot stage is also desirable to try out the questions, validate their use (i.e. check that they *do* measure what is wanted) and test whether they are answered reliably (i.e. that they produce the same answers when asked more than once). An important factor in questionnaire design is the avoidance of reactivity – the tendency for the pattern of the answers to be produced by the way the questions are asked rather than by genuine differences among informants. With more complex measuring scales pilot work is essential.

5 Surveys usually involve asking identical questions across a population, but more personalized explorations are also possible. Kelly's Role Repertory Grid is an example of an instrument designed for personalized exploration of beliefs and attitudes.

Further reading

Survey design

Hakim, Catherine (1987) *Research Design: Strategies and Choices in the Design of Social Research*. London: Routledge (Chapters 5, 7 and 8).

Oppenheim, A.N. (1992) *Questionnaire Design, Interviewing and Attitude Measurement*. London: Pinter (Chapters 1–4, 7–8).

Polgar, Stephen and Thomas, Shane (1988) *Introduction to Research in the Health Sciences*. London: Churchill Livingstone.

Witts, L.J. (ed.) (1964) *Medical Surveys and Clinical Trials*. London: Oxford University Press.

Measurement scales and psychological/attitude tests

Anastasi, Anne (1982) *Psychological Testing*. London: Macmillan.
Hollander, Edwin (1981) *Principles and Methods of Social Psychology*. Oxford: Oxford University Press (Chapter 3).
Jensen, Arthur (1981) *Straight Talk about Mental Tests*. London: Macmillan.
Newmark, Charles (1985) *Major Psychological Assessment Instruments*. Boston, MA: Allyn and Bacon.
Oppenheim, A.N. (1992) *Questionnaire Design, Interviewing and Attitude Measurement*. London: Pinter (Chapters 9–12).
Osgood, Charles, Sui, George and Tannenbaum, Percy (1967) *The Measurement of Meaning*. Urbana, IL: University of Illinois Press.

Role Repertory Grids and George Kelly's approach

Bannister, Don and Fransella, Fay (1980) *Inquiring Man*. Harmondsworth: Penguin.
Kelly, George (1955) *The Psychology of Personal Constructs*. New York: Norton.
Smith, Jonathan, Harre, Rom and Van Langenhove, Luk (1995) *Rethinking Methods in Social Psychology*. London: Sage (Chapter 11).

Quantitative (statistical) analysis

To teach statistics is beyond the scope of this book, but there are many good texts on the market. Two books are particularly recommended. The first is the best for the beginner, a very good introductory text; it was recommended to us by our students. The other is also good, and does not assume any prior knowledge of statistics, but it is pitched more at good third-year students and postgraduates.

Clegg, Frances (1982) *Simple Statistics*. Cambridge: Cambridge University Press.
Marsh, Catherine (1988) *Exploring Data*. Cambridge: Polity.

EXPERIMENTAL PRACTICE

In this chapter we shall assume that any **experiment** you want to carry out will be a 'field experiment', set in the real world. We shall look mainly at how you would go about evaluating some aspect of your own potential practice – how you would try out a new treatment technique or style of working. The same techniques would also be appropriate for wider-scale testing of new practices – for assessing the effects of a new management structure or a general change in practice imposed from outside, or for comparing wards or wings of an institution in which different regimes were in force. (You should note, however, that this kind of **controlled trial** is by no means the only way in which practices can be evaluated. Most of the rest of this book will be about evaluation, offering a wide range of styles of working. This chapter is firmly set within a positivist epistemology and is concerned more with demonstrating **causal** influences than with understanding the nature of phenomena.)

Uncontrolled trials

The simplest kind of 'experimental' research you can do is just 'trying things out' in its crudest form – making a change and seeing what happens. Though by no means the best design for the purpose, this is a very common form of research into practice, often used in circumstances where nothing more elaborate is possible or where insufficient preparation rules out better designs. Here we have termed it 'the *un*controlled trial' to distinguish it from more rigorously designed research. To obtain interpretable results, careful and **reliable** measurement and exhaustive documentation are essential. We need a clear and reliable measurement or description of what the treatment procedure or programme of change is, so that we know what it is that is causing any change that may occur. We need a clearly defined set of outcome measures, so that we can see what change is brought about. We need also to measure anything in the environment which might function as an alternative explanation of the results.

Measurement of the treatment and the outcome are not as simple as might at first appear. We need to have thought very carefully about what it is we are trying to achieve and what will count as having achieved it. In psychiatric and counselling research, for example, it is seldom possible to produce definitive proof of 'cure' following treatment – something that would be accepted by others, rather than just the researcher's/therapist's personal judgement. One tends, therefore, to ask the clients/patients what they *thought* of the therapy and whether they were satisfied with it; at least this is something more concrete than the therapist's judgement of his or her own cases. However, whether a feeling of satisfaction in the patient or client is what the therapist was trying to achieve is open to question: would he or she not be better satisfied with an amelioration of the condition, whether or not the patient felt good about the therapy. There is a great tendency in experimental research to substitute something measurable but not totally appropriate for the outcome which we really want to assess. If you were carrying out the research for someone else, you would need to think even more carefully about what outcome is desired and not necessarily to accept what the client said was the outcome. A declared aim of a hospital administration, for example, might be to improve the care of certain patients, as measured perhaps by whether they had to be readmitted for the same condition within a specified time period. However, it is a reasonable bet that they would not implement a recommendation to increase staffing levels unless it could be shown that the costs of readmission were higher than those of increasing the intensity of nursing care.

Reactivity is the second problem. Inevitably, your ideas about the measurement of effectiveness have an effect on your practice – you do such and such because it appears to be working. We have hinted at this already, talking about problems in defining output measures: it is essential that you define what shall count as a success *before* starting to measure. Otherwise you are in the position of the punter who placed his bet after the race was won: you are claiming to predict what you have, in fact, observed happening. The nature of the treatment itself is even more prone to reactive effects in this kind of research. To the extent that you are not able to define precisely what your treatment will be *before* starting to measure its effects, your results will always be suspect: you may always have modified what you are doing to fit in with changes which you have observed (unconsciously, even). There will also be **confounded variables** – factors associated with your treatment which might provide alternative explanations of the outcome. In the earlier part of this century, great claims were made for the efficacy of insulin injections as a cure for certain kinds of mental disorder. These claims were dispelled by later analysis of what the process entailed – extreme physical debilitation, followed during the recovery period by constant and sympathetic attention from nurses. The subsequent discovery that the attention and sympathy were equally effective when *not* accompanied by the insulin injection more or less put paid to this therapy's claims.

The problem is in three parts:

1 There will be aspects to what you are doing of which you are not aware, probably aspects of your own behaviour and the way you budget your time.
2 These may as easily explain any changes which you observe as the deliberate manipulation of treatment which you are instituting.
3 There may be no way, within the crude design of this kind of research, of separating out these effects: doing a certain kind of therapy or social work or nursing care may inevitably mean spending more time with the 'experimental' subjects or behaving to them in a certain kind of way, and it may always be this rather than the deliberate manipulation which is producing the effect.

The best you can do is to try to note all these confounded influences, perhaps, if possible, getting someone else to watch you at work and examine your practice – and note them in your report as areas for further study.

Exercise 30: Critique of uncontrolled trials

Imagine you have just joined the staff of a ward or office where a new procedure has been introduced. What steps would you take to monitor its progress? (Assume that back records, etc. are not available.) More important, what could you *not* conclude from your results? (Think of this as a logical problem, not a practical one.)

However well you design this kind of study, it has certain logical flaws which inevitably mean that what can be concluded from it is strictly limited. You may institute a change and observe a result. However:

1 you can never be quite sure what produced the result – all manner of things will have been changed by the fact of your instituting an 'experiment', apart from your nominated treatment or experimental manipulation;
2 there may have been differences between people which are equally responsible for who showed the 'effect', and while you may have collected information about these, your 'sample' will lack sufficient structure for you to be able to disentangle or disprove such effects by statistical means;
3 you will not be able to say whether the effect would have occurred even without the treatment;
4 worst of all, you will not even be able to specify what the effect is – you will have measurements on how people perform after the treatment, but in the design discussed so far you have nothing with which to compare them.

Towards the controlled trial

The easiest of the faults to remedy in this very crude research design is the problem of knowing whether a change has occurred or not. The first and most basic element in any experimental design is that measurement of the **dependent variable**(s) shall be undertaken *before* the manipulation/treatment is undertaken as well as afterwards. Indeed, to do so would be characteristic of any decently planned **action research**. Your basic data, in looking for causal influences, are not measurements, but differences between measurements: we are looking, not for some absolute value of a dependent variable, but for a change in it. You might, indeed, go further: if what you have achieved is a lasting change, not just a temporary one, then you will need post-treatment measurements after a period of time to demonstrate the fact.

However, a series of measurements on one group which has received a treatment are not in themselves logically convincing. Certainly, you can demonstrate that a change has occurred, but you cannot demonstrate *why* it occurred. Specifically, you cannot demonstrate that it occurred as a result of the treatment which was applied; it may be due to any number of other things which occurred to the group being treated during the same time as the treatment. The other essential of experimental design, therefore, is a **control** or **comparison group** – one which is alike in every respect to the treatment group, and undergoes as similar as possible a set of experiences, but does not actually receive the treatment. (In drug research they would typically receive a placebo or dummy – a pill or injection which looked like the experimental drug but was in fact chemically inert.) One basic stratagem for making sure that the two groups are alike is to assign people randomly to treatment and control groups, as we have seen: provided your groups are reasonably large, this should 'even out' any chance differences. Guaranteeing similarity of experience is more difficult, outside the laboratory, but you would want to document their lives in as much detail as possible during the period of the experiment, looking for any possibly significant differences.

As we pointed out in Chapter 5, there are other ways of picking control/comparison groups which may be more effective for some purposes. With small numbers you probably need to institute some kind of **matching** procedure, picking pairs of subjects who are comparable on variables which you know might well be important (age, class, gender, medical condition, social circumstances, or whatever) and allocating one of the pair at random to each group. This absolutely guarantees comparability at least on these variables. Indeed, where you are trying to control for some well known alternative explanation at the design stage, matching is perhaps the best stratagem; like **stratification** in **random sampling** (see Chapter 9), it may improve on the simple random procedures in ways which are important to you. Best of all, if your design lends itself to it, is to use the same subjects as both 'experimentals' and 'controls': then you are certain that those in the two groups have the same history, the same physical and mental constitution, etc. This is seldom possible in practice, however, because the administration of the treatment alters the subjects to the point where they are no longer comparable with their past selves with regard to the manipulation which you want to test.

The allocation of subjects to treatment and control groups raises an important point about the conduct of experiments. It is for each researcher to decide whether the purity of including an untreated control group is worth the ethical dilemma of leaving some people deliberately untreated, but on the whole many researchers and professionals would regard doing so as unethical in a wide range of circumstances. A way round may be to compare a new treatment with people undergoing the best of what was previously available: then at least no one has deliberately been debarred from treatment. It is often difficult to reconcile the needs of the research – including the benefit to future sufferers if a treatment can be shown unambiguously to 'work' – with the deliberate mis- or non-treatment of a proportion of sufferers.

A final point to watch is what is known as the Hawthorne Effect (a form of reactivity). The name derives from a famous series of studies at the Hawthorne Works in Chicago in the 1920s (Roethlisberger and Dickson 1939). The researchers were commissioned to seek ways of changing environment and working conditions to improve output, and they tried out a range of possible modifications, each of which did, indeed, improve output – improving lighting and physical comfort, introducing coffee breaks, shortening the working day, etc. However, when as the last stage of the experiment (using a 'same-subjects' design) they returned everything to its original state, output went up again. It was concluded that the major (and confounded) variable, which might have been responsible for any of the results, was the subjects' awareness that they were taking part in an experiment. To the extent that the subjects of your treatment know that it is a new treatment, their reactions may be conditioned by this knowledge as much as by the treatment itself. Even your own knowledge that your treatment is experimental may change your behaviour in unconscious ways: how you behave may not be how you would behave if the new procedure had been accepted and you were applying it routinely. Drug researchers commonly adopt what is called a **double-blind** technique, where neither the recipient of the drug nor the person handing it out in conformity with a prearranged administration schedule knows whether what is received is the active drug or an inactive placebo. The ethics of this kind of procedure in social research may again be open to question, however.

Exercise 31: Experiment

Try making some small change in your own practice: a change of procedures or the ordering of jobs, aimed at getting patients to talk to each other more, or a different way of arranging your interviews with people to set them apparently more at their ease, or a different way of budgeting your time to allow more time for study or to get the household chores over faster. Think carefully, before you start, what precisely your manipulation or treatment is to be – write it out as a set of instructions for yourself – and what is to count as having achieved your desired outcome (in measurable terms). Think what other changes might occur as a result of your changed behaviour, which might affect the outcome, and think about ways of measuring these and controlling for them either in the design or by **statistical control** at the stage of analysis. Start your measurements before you start your 'treatment', to give yourself a baseline 'before' measure with which your outcome can be compared. Think carefully also about the extent to which the fact that it is your own practice which you are examining may contaminate the results. For example, to what extent might the awareness of an impending experimental change affect your behaviour during the period of measurement before the experiment started?

Single-case experimental designs

Schematically, this kind of design can be represented as ABA or perhaps ABlB2B3A – untreated state (A) followed by treatment (B) followed by a period of untreated observation (A), or perhaps untreated state (A) followed by a series of treatments until one appears to work (B1, B2, B3 . . .), followed by a period of observation without treatment (A). The problem is in establishing the **validity** of the conclusion that it is the treatment (or something associated with it) which produces the effect. As a logical argument this form of study is obviously weak: it lacks the evidence of the same procedure working on several different people, and it lacks any element of **replication** – repeating it to see if it works twice (with the inference that if it does not work the second time then the first effect may have been a fluke). The basic form of any superstitious argument lies in an appeal to this kind of experience (I crossed my fingers and the terrible thing failed to happen, so it must not have happened because I crossed my fingers – ignoring the many times when one has crossed one's fingers without effect, and the many times that something terrible has happened and might well have happened even if one did cross one's fingers).

A basic element of the single-case experimental design is measurement over time and the comparison of treatment with the state of the subject while untreated. Thus the simplest kind of project would establish baseline measurements before treatment and then alternate application and withdrawal of treatment – ABABABA . . . In this way the subject acts as 'control' as well as 'treatment' condition – the state when untreated repeatedly acts as a comparison point for the state after treatment. There is variability within subjects as well as between them – people differ across time – but by alternating treatments one effectively controls for within-subject variability. It is possible to evaluate different treatments against each other by this means as well, comparing each with the untreated state – ABlAB2AB3 . . . (Because the person changes in the course of the treatment series, it would actually be necessary to apply each several times in alternation – ABlAB2ABlAB2 . . .) The argument always rests on the stability of Condition A, the untreated condition, however; the subject may show variation, but this must average out. The basic 'resting state' against which all else is compared must broadly resemble itself from one period of measurement to another (or any trends must be calculable, so that allowance can be made for them).

A second way of overcoming the variability of the individual subject is by frequently repeated measurement. If you were working with a group of subjects you would take a measurement from each of them and average them to get a stable estimate of how the group was proceeding. With the single subject this is not possible, so one has to average over time, which means measurement at more frequent intervals than would be normal in group research. The measurements can then be added together and averaged to give a single reading for a designated time-period; this is to some extent free of chance variation because several different readings have gone into it, any of which could by chance have varied in either direction from the average. Repeated measurement over a reasonably long time-period is particularly important at the diagnostic stage, to establish with some reliability the baseline against which the results of treatment(s) are to be judged.

The problem with single-case designs, quite clearly, is establishing validity, reliability and generality without the power to average between subjects to eliminate chance fluctuations and unique events. Repeated and frequent measurement may answer the problem of reliability – the extent to which the measures taken are stable ones – by the direct test of repeating them. Validity may be established by a number of means: validity of measurement by using already validated tests, or by using more than one observer or more than one kind of measure and checking that all show similar trends; validity of design by careful specification of the treatment and careful definition of goals, and by putting great care into establishing that the initial baseline measurements are stable. The question of generalizability is more difficult; it is difficult to generalize from the single subject to a population. Sometimes, where the aim is assessing the results of a particular therapy on the single patient, this may not matter. Often, however, one wishes to be able to say whether a treatment that has succeeded in this case would succeed in others, and if so, then which others. The best we can do here is to argue that what works for one subject stands a reasonable chance of working with other 'similar' subjects. Single-case research may be a good way of building techniques, but research on groups may be needed to test them.

We have stressed the disadvantages of single-case studies, in terms of generalizability. One should realize, however, that there are countervailing disadvantages to studies of groups. The need in **applied research** to work with what is available may lead to very unrepresentative group results; where a 'problem' is not randomly spread through the population, and where a non-random subsection of those coming forward with it actually reaches research attention, there is no reason to suppose that an available group is any more **representative** of the population than a single case. Indeed, because of the depth in which single cases are studied and the effort which is put into specifying the population of which they may be **typical**, it can in practice be true that single-case research is more readily generalizable than more conventional research carried out on groups.

The generality of results from single-case research is . . . a major issue. Concerns often have been voiced about the fact that only one or two subjects are studied at a time and the extent to which findings extend to other persons is not known. Actually, there is no evidence that findings from single-case research are any less generalisable than findings from between-group research. In fact, because of the type of interventions studied in single-case research, the case is sometimes made that the results may be more generalisable than those obtained in between-group research.

(Kazdin 1982: 288)

A major check on results, in single-case research as in any other, is replication – doing the job again. In probability terms, if the probability of a chance result is low when you do the research once, then the chances multiply when you do it twice and get the same result. The chance of drawing the King of Spades from the pack once is 1 in 52. The chances of doing so twice are 1 in $52 \times 52 = 2704$ – vanishingly small. Where there are doubts of generalizability and of control of sporadic variation, as in single-case designs, replication becomes particularly important. It is for this reason that the ABAB design is seen as basic to single-case research – it builds in one automatic replication on the same case. Partial and systematic replication may be used to explore conceptually distinct aspects of the original successful treatment, by varying aspects of the original 'package' systematically in subsequent cases.

Replication can be accomplished in different ways depending on the precise aspect of generality in which the investigator is interested. To investigate generality across subjects, the investigator can conduct a direct replication . . . applying the same procedures across a number of different subjects. To evaluate the generality of findings across a variety of different conditions . . . the investigator can conduct a systematic replication . . . purposely allowing features of the original experiment to vary . . . Actually, direct and systematic replications are not qualitatively different. An exact replication is not possible in principle since repetition of the experiment involves new subjects tested at different points of time and perhaps by different investigators . . . all replications necessarily allow some factors to vary.

(Kazdin 1982: 284)

Exercise 32: Planning a single-case experimental design

Develop a plan for research into the treatment of obesity in a single patient. How would you demonstrate validity, reliability and generalizability? What modifications might you need to make to render your design ethically acceptable as research?

There are no right answers to these questions, but our attempts at them may be found at the end of the chapter.

Quasi-experimental logic

A sure way of getting over most ethical problems with experimental research is the **natural experiment** or **quasi-experimental** comparison (the **case-control study** of medical research). Here what you do is to take a change which is being imposed anyway and collect or obtain statistics from before the change, during it and after it. These are treated as the 'pre-test' and 'post-test' statistics of the true experiment. You can generally organize some kind of control or comparison group as well: a similar area in which the change is not occurring, for example. A classic example is the Connecticut Crackdown, a change in motoring laws in one American state which was aimed at decreasing traffic fatalities. A team of researchers looked at the changes it made to fatality statistics by comparing figures from before the changes of law and practice to figures from after it (Campbell and Ross 1968; Ross and Campbell 1968; Campbell 1969). They controlled for extraneous events by comparing surrounding states, where these changes had not been made, and found that fatalities did not decrease similarly over the same period. The argument that it was the changes in law and practice which brought about the change in death-rate is, therefore, fairly convincing, and the logic of the argument follows the argument of an experiment. Its weakness, however, is that the design is not experimental in that there is no control over allocation to experimental and control groups. However carefully the two are matched, it is always possible to argue that there may be some unobserved difference between the two which is responsible for the results.

Finally, two points which we have made earlier in the book are worth repeating here, because they have implications for your own design of research:

1 The basic purpose of many pieces of **survey** research is quasi-experimental comparison – looking for the association of one variable with another, with the intention of arguing about causal influence. This is why it is so important to pre-guess alternative explanations and collect variables relevant to them, to be able to eliminate them by statistical control at the analysis stage.

2 On the other hand, many studies which masquerade as true experiments are at best quasi-experimental, because there is no true control over allocation to groups. Experiments comparing males and females, for example, are at best quasi-experimental: there may be characteristics contingently associated with gender but not central to its definition – such as experience of early socialization, for example, or outright discrimination and stereotyping in adult life – which are confounded with gender itself and cannot be eliminated by any kind of random allocation. The same holds true for experiments comparing clinical types, or different types of offender, or any experiments where the allocation to groups rests in essence on a 'naturally' occurring difference.

Summary

1 The simplest kind of 'experimental' research which you can do, which we have called 'the uncontrolled trial' involves making a change and looking to see what follows. This is badly flawed as a design, because it does not compare the outcome with the 'state of play' *before* the change was made, so it is not possible to say with certainty that any change *did* occur.

2 A true experiment (or 'controlled trial') involves measurement before the change, the imposition of a change on one group but not another, measurement after the change, and so a demonstration that a difference occurred as a result of the change in the group which was 'treated' but not in the other group. If the two groups differed in nothing except the experimental treatment, then this design is a very strong demonstration of the causal effect of the treatment.

3 Clear and unambiguous measurement of **independent variable** (treatment), **dependent variables** (effects) and other variables on which the groups might have differed before or during treatment is essential for this kind of research.

4 It is possible to run experiments on single cases. They generally involve repeated measurements and the imposition of one or more treatments according to a controlled and logical pattern.

5 There are often very serious ethical problems involved in experimental research, to do with the manipulation of subjects against their interests or the withholding of treatment from some subjects in order to form a control group.

6 Quasi-experimental analysis can be carried out with a similar degree of rigour in logic and measurement on changes which are occurring 'naturally' in the world. This avoids many of the ethical problems of the experiment. It is never possible, however, to demonstrate with rigour that it was the treatment and not something else which produced the effect.

Further reading

Breakwell, Glynnis, Foot, Hugh and Gilmour, Robin (eds) (1982) *Social Psychology: A Practical Manual*. London: Macmillan/British Psychological Society.

Hakim, Catherine (1987) *Research Design: Strategies and Choices in the Design of Social Research*. London: Routledge (Chapter 9).

Hersen, Michael and Barlow, David (1976) *Single-case Experimental Designs*. Oxford: Pergamon.

Kazdin, Alan (1982) *Single-case Research Designs*. Oxford: Oxford University Press.

Polgar, Stephen and Thomas, Shane (1988) *Introduction to Research in the Health Sciences*. London: Churchill Livingstone.

Witts, L.J. (ed.) (1964) *Medical Surveys and Clinical Trials*. London: Oxford University Press.

Answer to Exercise 32

What you would do here depends crucially on your theoretical stance. If you are taking a behavioural stance to the problem, you would be focusing on overeating as a set of habits and looking for weight reduction via control of eating or control of circumstances in which eating takes place. Your 'treatment' might involve making the person aware of how much he or she eats, and how often, by getting him or her to keep a 'food diary' and even perhaps to weigh all food before eating. It might involve a controlled diet, to reaccustom the stomach to being less distended. It might involve identifying the circumstances under which the person 'snacks' and getting him or her to avoid those circumstances, or substituting another activity – walking, listening to music – for the snacking. If you take a more **holistic** stance you might be looking more to underlying factors which initiate the overeating – depression or over-strain or some idea of making oneself more or less attractive for some at most half-admitted purpose. Then your treatment might involve counselling – to attack the feelings and self-judgements directly – and an attempt to rearrange the person's life to make it more rewarding or to substitute other rewards for the rewards of eating.

Whichever, the first stage would have to be a very thorough investigation of the existing situation – how heavy the person is and how the weight fluctuates, what is eaten and when, what the person does during the day, with whom (and with what success) he or she interacts, what demands are placed on him or her, perhaps his or her self-image and beliefs about the self, and his or her feelings and beliefs about food and eating. A goal would be formulated in terms of weight loss and perhaps a change in patterns of social interaction. (The goals would have to be formulated in collaboration with the client – ethically because it is his or her body and his or her life, and practically because the client would be the one actually to 'apply the treatment'.) You would arrange for the client to keep records during the treatment, and times would be assigned for you to visit again to collect information yourself. At regular intervals you would monitor the achievement of the goals and decide whether to discontinue the 'treatment', to continue with it or to change it, and to see whether other problems emerged apart from the one you were 'treating'. At the end, after treatment is discontinued, you would continue to monitor for a while, to ensure that progress was maintained.

You would deliberately alternate periods of treatment and non-treatment – return to previous behaviour – to establish convincingly that it was the treatment that produced the effect. You might well feel that this kind of experiment, with its deliberate reversions to the untreated condition, was not an ethically justified way of proceeding against any problem which really mattered to the client, whether or not consent and collaboration was achieved.

OPEN INTERVIEWING

This chapter deals with the conduct of 'open' or 'unstructured' interviews with groups of people. You might be interviewing simply to find out people's views on a topic or a service, not knowing enough in advance to put together a structured **questionnaire**. (Indeed, a short phase of open interviewing is a normal precursor to constructing a questionnaire – 'mapping the ground', finding out the range of views and topics which should be covered, learning the language in which informants are likely to express themselves.) You might be exploring a topic where it is desirable not to introduce previous theory, but to 'let the participants speak for themselves'. Much feminist work is of this kind, trying not to apply preconceived (and male-conceived) categories to women's lives, but talking to them to see what they think is important and how they understand their world. You might be carrying out an evaluation of a setting or of a service you have been providing, and need to get at how the clients and staff have experienced it without letting your own or management's preconceptions intrude. You might be doing something much less structured – talking to groups of people in categories of interest, just to understand their lives and how they make sense of them.

'Open interviewing' is not one method, but our term for a range of different ways of proceeding. They have in common:

1 the aim of eliciting the informants' views in the informants' own terms;
2 the attempt to make the interviews resemble natural conversations as far as possible;
3 the desire to impose as little as possible of the researchers' ideas on the conversation.

While agreeing on these aims, however, interviewers have differed a great deal over how to pursue them. Some interviews are virtually undirected by the researcher, with the informant controlling most of the direction of the conversation. In others the interviewers take more control, trying to cut through 'irrelevance' and 'keeping the informant to the point'. Most interviewers go in with an outline 'agenda', but for some this consists only of a list of topic areas to cover and a few 'stock questions' to get things started and bridge gaps in the conversation. In other cases, however, the researcher may have a quite detailed list of questions to ask of all informants and may even try to determine the order in which they are answered. Mostly, we adopt a 'neutrally sympathetic' manner when interviewing, but in some research (e.g. on managers of large corporations) the researchers have thought it appropriate to adopt an adversarial style and provoke an argument in order to test the informants' beliefs. All of these are valid ways of doing interview research, and each has its strengths and corresponding weaknesses. On the whole, the more structured the approach, the less the **naturalism** and the more the danger of attributing the researchers' ideas to the informants. On the other hand, structure makes for uniformity of coverage and so for more interpretable data.

After an initial section on kinds of design for interview projects we work backwards in this chapter, from the nature of the work to the ways in which it is conducted. What kind of an exercise you think you are undertaking – what model you hold of the informants and their social world – shapes not only the analysis of the data, but also the conduct of the interviews and the way the study is initially planned, so this is considered first. Thereafter, we talk about the conduct of interviews, about gaining access to informants and about the selection of informants.

Life-history interviews and comparative interviewing

One form of open interviewing is the 'life-history interview', where you pick a single informant and interview repeatedly, exploring the whole of his or her life. You would start off in a comparatively non-directive fashion – perhaps making sure that each segment of the life was covered, and redirecting the informant from what were obviously long and non-productive detours, but otherwise asking little except 'What happened next?' In later interviews you might want to clarify the earlier ones – we are all sometimes inconsistent and even inaccurate in detailing our past lives, and the 'outside eye' of an interviewer can often help to clarify chronology – and to feed back reports of later judgements which are formally inconsistent with reports of earlier ones (as where a particular person is reported as untrustworthy in describing an early stage of life but as a friend in a later one or vice versa). In still later interviews you will be questioning expressed value judgements, to make sure you understand them and their limitations, and posing formal inconsistencies as questions for the informant to rethink. In later interviews again you might be posing the questions which matter to you as a researcher/practitioner.

Life-history interviewing allows a considerable penetration into informants' lives as they see them and gives access to the unobservable past (though necessarily refocused through the lens of the present – present views and concerns shape our memories and our understanding of our own past lives). Most open interviewing contains some element of life-history work; it is a very good technique for getting people talking about their lives in their own words and concepts, without imposing the views and concepts of the researcher. However, a single informant is a limited field for generalization, and most open interviewing involves interviews with a larger number – perhaps ten or 20 informants. With larger numbers it is possible to introduce a comparative element, comparing the views of women with men, for example, or practitioners with patients, or those to whom some event has happened with otherwise similar people to whom it has not. This kind of comparison draws on the same logic as that of the **experiment** and is essential for bounded generalization. You cannot, for example, say what is true of women as opposed to men – how the genders differ – from interviews with women alone; you need a basis of comparison.

Open interviewing of one informant or groups of informants is the approach which you would undoubtedly use if your field of study were not already well researched, or if you were unhappy with the research and theorization which dominated the field so far. It allows you to carry out research which is **holistic** and comparatively unfocused. That is, it does not focus in on variables, but tries for a complete description of the person's life and how he or she sees the social world. Within this description you hope to find your 'problem' – health attitudes, or growing old and coping, or dealing with heart disease in the family – located and intermeshed with all the other aspects of life and relationship. (If not, a bit of judicious probing will undoubtedly allow you to trace out the relationships.) Even if you propose a **survey** or **experiment** at a later date, in an ill-explored field you would undoubtedly start with some form of open, qualitative interviewing, and life-history interviewing is the form which imposes least structure and preconception on the informant.

It may also be a relevant way of conducting research into practice. What we have talked about so far are treatment-oriented techniques of differing degrees of **reductionism** and quantitative complexity. Another kind of evaluation of the service you are providing, however, stands back from immediate detail and tries to understand the client's or patient's life as a whole, with your treatment-oriented concerns fading to become just one part, and perhaps not a very large part. Understanding maternity, or old age, or chronic disability or the problems of those caring for sick or disabled dependants might best be approached by this means. It might also give you a better perspective than more focused evaluation on whether the service you provide is effective, or relevant, or even noticed particularly by the informant. More focused evaluation techniques can explore treatment packages and service provision in the terms in which you conceive them, but to explore their place in the informant's life you need the more open and less prestructured approach which open interviewing can offer.

The disadvantage – or indeed, perhaps the advantage – of this approach to understanding the informant's life is that it is almost entirely retrospective. You are asking the informant to tell the story of his or her life from now backwards, or from the beginning until now, but in either case it will be told as it makes sense now. It will be an account from the point of view of the present, weighted according to present concerns and structured to make sense of the present. The informant may on occasion be able to report that 'things seemed different then', but even this is an account of past feeling structured from the point of view of the present. The disadvantage, as with all accounts, is that the past will be 'constructed' to make sense. (This is not because it is the past, but because what we have is an account; an account of the present would be similarly constructed to make sense.) The advantage is that what we learn is not an array of dispassionate 'facts', but that way of structuring the informant's past which demonstrates (or conceals, but makes available for discovery) its impact on present life and attitudes.

Exercise 33: Life history and comparative interviewing

If you were exploring the theme of obesity, how would you go about conducting a life-history interview to cast light on the topic? What sort of person would you want as informant? How would you approach the task and structure the series of interviews? Under what circumstances might the outcome be relevant for professional practice?

    What could a series of comparative interviews tell you that life-history interviewing of a single informant could not? Where might the life-history interviews be *more* informative?

    Our attempts at answers are at the end of the chapter.

The nature of the data

At its simplest, the open interview is a way of finding out what people *think* about a situation. With the minimum of imposed structure necessary to keep the focus of the interview within bounds and save ourselves the time involved in listening to totally extraneous material, we let people talk about the situation and what matters to them about it. This is by far the best way of finding out what is *salient* to them about it – what most readily springs to their lips. With a little probing to get them to assess which ideas matter and which are just 'tried on' to see how well they hold together in the interview situation, we can assess what is *central* – what they see as the irreducible core of their beliefs. We would probably impose an agenda of areas to be covered, so that we can be sure all informants have covered the same ground. We should be careful how we used such an agenda, however, or our introduction of particular topics could obscure whether they were, in fact, salient for the particular informant; once we have introduced a topic, we can no longer tell whether it would have cropped up spontaneously in the course of the interview.

An alternative view of how people work and make sense of their world is to see them as not always aware of what is important to them. If we want to know what the informant *feels* – what motivates his or her behaviour, whether or not he or she is aware of it or able (or willing) to mobilize it in conversation – then we must see our task in a rather different way. People may well have a set of well articulated views – a '**rhetoric**' – which are strongly held and firmly believed, but their actual behaviour and the decisions they make may sometimes suggest to the outsider a quite different set of norms and values. For example, the more educated respondents generally have a clear and consistent set of beliefs to enunciate about social class, the structure of society and their place in it. When it comes to asking them about the detail of their lives, however – which schools their children go to and why they are 'good' or 'bad', which areas they see as good or bad ones to live in and why, what kinds of job they wish for their children and why – an equally clear set of implicit beliefs often emerges, but one which is not consistent with their declared 'rhetorical' position. This matter of rhetoric is an important one for open interviewing: whether we accept what the informant says at face value, or allow that we may all have sets of verbal beliefs which are sincerely held but which may not be the unifying principles behind our practical actions.

If you hold this view of how people work in the social world, then you will be imposing a little more structure on the occasion than if you just accept what informants say at face value. You will be introducing questions, and areas of discussion, precisely in order to 'get underneath' the rhetoric and see what you can elicit about the less formally organized and recognized structuring principles which people apply to the social world when making their practical decisions. Doing so, however, will face you with the ethical question of the extent to which you are prepared to 'lead informants on' in order to elicit from them material which it is your intention to interpret in ways which might well offend them.

Now suppose that what you are trying to find out is what the informants *want done about* a situation – how to solve a problem which has occurred, or how to improve an institutional setting, say. A mixture of these two models would undoubtedly be what is appropriate. You would be required and require yourself to represent faithfully the views which the participants had expressed. At the same time you might suspect that the immediate focus of complaint was not really 'what was wrong', and so you would be looking beyond and underneath their 'rhetoric' for more nebulous features of their situation which might be at fault. If you were playing your research to any extent **collaboratively** – as seems wise and reasonable, if there were any chance of your 'solution' being foisted on the informants – then you would want to discuss your eventual conclusions with them and reshape them to reflect their reactions (perhaps several times, until you found a set of recommendations and a form of words for expressing them which was acceptable to all parties). Given courage, you might even discuss your conclusions about particular interviews with the individual participants, before coming to a public set of general conclusions. This would take courage, however, if you had presumed to any extent to 'see behind the words' and draw conclusions on the basis of knowing better than the informant what was important in his or her life.

Doing the interviews

The core of the open style of interviewing is a very lively appreciation of how you are trying to present yourself and the task, and the way in which the informant is making sense of the task and of you (in a word, **reflexivity**).

Right from the start of any such project you would be watching carefully whether you 'came across' in your professional identity (social worker, nurse, doctor), or as a student, or as a researcher perhaps associated with an academic institution, or as someone writing a book, or whatever. You will be monitoring carefully the impression you give of the task – whether it is a student exercise, or the gratification of your own curiosity, or an academic investigation, or a study of shortcomings that might perhaps be put right as a result of it. Who you are and what the task is seen to be is all the informants have out of which to make sense of the exercise, and what sense they make will crucially determine what kind of an account they give of the phenomena in which you are interested.

Your choice of location for the interview (if you have a choice!) will be governed by the principle of naturalism: you will try to put yourself and the interview in a 'frame' which might be a natural one for the informant. For many purposes the informant's own home may be the best setting – putting oneself in the territory of the other – but there are circumstances where the home might be the wrong context. Talking to people about their work, for instance, it may be better to talk at the workplace or, better still, wherever they go to relax after work sessions – the canteen, the staff room, the local public house. There may be circumstances where the interview is best conducted on your own territory – in your office, or at the hospital bedside – but this will generally be appropriate only if you normally ask questions or have conversations with that informant in that setting. Best of all, if you are doing more than one interview with the same person, may be to vary the setting and take note of the different shades of perspective which are expressed in the different settings.

In the interview itself you will be trying to present yourself as friendly but neutral, as someone not intimately involved in any disputes or differences of interest which may be mentioned. If the conversation is to be at all natural and relaxed you will have to say a bit about yourself and to contribute opinions to the flow of the occasion. To the extent that it is possible, however, you will avoid doing so – even if you are adopting a collaborative stance and interviewing for a declared and agreed purpose. It is all too easy, reading the transcript of an interview after the event, to see where opinions or categorizations of your own have been taken up and incorporated by the informant, so that you cannot tell whether they are part of the way in which the informant sees the world or on loan from the interviewer. It is regrettably all too easy to express your own attitude to a situation and have the respondent agree with you – perhaps out of conviction, but perhaps out of politeness or a desire to adopt a 'socially desirable point of view'. Insofar as is possible, in a situation which can only be what it is because of your participation in it, you must avoid these forms of **reactivity** by contributing as little as you can; it is the informant whose views and feelings you want to collect, not your own. To the extent that detachment is not possible, you must try to be aware of your own contribution, take notes on it immediately afterwards, and if necessary report on it in your account of the findings.

Before entering the field you will have taken the opportunity to read as much as you can about the background and circumstances of the people whom you will be interviewing. If you are to be working in a hospital, you will read anything that has been written on that hospital or that class of hospitals, including what is said about it in Parliament and in the newspapers, to get a feel for the 'working rules' and the declared aims, and to be aware of any outstanding problems (e.g. financial). If you are interviewing a particular class of professional staff, you will scan their professional journals for articles expressing their problems and discontents and for what you can find on the letter page. If you are talking to a group of people who have a given medical condition, you will familiarize yourself with the literature on that condition. If you are talking to people who fall in a 'social problem' category, you will make sure you are familiar with the benefits and services available to such a group. When you go into the field you will want to be as well informed as possible, so that you do not miss veiled allusions to common features of the situation and so that you are aware of any glaring omissions in participants' accounts.

On the other hand, you will want to conceal your knowledge as far as possible. The correct role for the qualitative researcher has often been described as that of the 'amiable incompetent' – someone friendly and intelligent but lacking knowledge, someone who has to be *told* things. (This may pose ethical problems, when for instance you know of some benefit or service to which the informant is entitled, but which he or she has not claimed. Try to restrict the information which you yourself communicate to the end of interviews, so as not to contaminate the material you collect or to 'break role' more than is necessary.)

Two particular problems arise when you are yourself a known 'expert', e.g. a health visitor interviewing other health visitors. The first is that it is difficult to get your informants to 'spell things out', because they assume you must know all about it already. The other and more serious is that you will find it difficult to put aside your professional socialization and 'make the familiar strange' – to ask your informants to spell out what they mean rather than filling in the gaps from your own knowledge. This matters because your knowledge may, in fact, be faulty: informants may not mean what you take for granted that they mean, and they may not have shared precisely your professional experience.

How much you ask direct questions will depend on the time available and the subject of the interview. To get the best out of this approach you will want at least some early portion of the interview to be conducted in a fairly undirected fashion, letting the informant develop things at his or her pace and seeing what crops up without prompting. To be sure you have covered the topic which is of interest to you in enough detail that you can be sure of doing justice to your informant's views, however, you may have to resort to direct prompting, to explore topic areas that have not come up by themselves. Remember, however, that once a topic has been introduced by you, you can never know whether it would have come up spontaneously. Best practice if time permits might be to have more than one interview with each informant and to save direct prompts for later ones; then you could also introduce questions on views and topic areas which had not come up in the particular interview but *had* been raised by another informant.

Selecting informants

While **representative** sampling is not and cannot be a major issue in this kind of work, because the sample size you will be able to handle is small, there is nonetheless every reason to try to pick 'cases' **randomly** from a sampling frame if at all possible, to avoid the charge of having deliberately chosen them to make a point or of having an unrealized bias in the sampling. In our mental handicap research (Abbott and Sapsford 1987b), for example, we were able to use the rolls of the 'special schools' as a sampling frame for families with a mentally handicapped child. There was no similar frame for the comparison group of families with no child bearing this label, however. What we did was to ask each interviewed mother for names and addresses of two or three other women on the same street or nearby who had a child of about the same chronological age as the mentally handicapped child, and how many other children they had. This enabled us to pick a comparison group who were roughly **matched** on geographical location (which was related to social class) and number of children. (We did not ask for introductions, preferring to make our own.) Sometimes personal introduction is the only way to put together a group for interview at all, if the criterion characteristic is a rare or concealed one – asking one example for names of others, asking them for further names, and continuing in this way until a sufficiently large group of interviews is achieved. This process is called **snowball sampling**, and it risks the obvious biases that you will only have access to 'cases' who know other 'cases', not to isolates, and that you may exhaust one part of the 'field' without ever encountering the other part. For example, in the mental handicap research a snowball sample which started with a mother whose child was at one type of special school might have given us a group of mothers from that school and none from the other school (which would have mattered, as the two schools dealt with cases of different severity). However, it may, on occasion, be the only way of proceeding.

A characteristic of an extended open interview project design is often the use of **theoretical sampling** – the selection of cases and groups, initially or as the research progresses, to explore aspects of the developing conclusions. In the mental handicap research, for example, we knew from the start that we would want to interview mothers of 'ordinary' children as well as mothers of mentally handicapped ones, to be able to distinguish problems of having a handicapped child from the general problems of having a child at all. If time and resources had allowed the research to continue further, we might have interviewed a group of mothers of physically handicapped children (to distinguish problems of *mental* handicap), or perhaps families caring for mentally handicapped adults (to distinguish problems associated with mentally handicapped *children*).

Gaining access

We have mentioned already the problem of 'gatekeepers'. Often it is necessary to get past certain key figures before gaining access to the informants whom you want to interview. In a hospital you would need the permission of the administrative authorities, the cooperation of those in charge of wards and of other nursing staff, probably clearance from an Ethical Committee, and so on. At each of these stages three things will be happening. First, you will be giving an account of your research, and this will undoubtedly be passed on, if only in a spirit of helpfulness and to prepare the ground for you. Your initial introduction to the setting will, therefore, be made not by you but by the gatekeepers. The second is that by having the permission or active cooperation of those in authority you may become identified with them in the eyes of the informants – particularly important in prison or school research, or in any setting where informants feel themselves controlled. You can do a certain amount to counteract these effects in your own initial introduction and in the course of the interviews, but you need to be alert for any differences they may have made to how you are perceived and what kinds of account you are being given. Such circumstances might be seen as a very good reason for interviewing each informant more than once, to try and build up an independent relationship of your own with them. The third effect will be that gatekeepers control to some extent whom you interview, steering you away from those who in their judgement are likely to be disturbed or harmed by the process. They may even steer you away from 'awkward cases' who would, in fact, make perfectly good informants, because in their judgement these people would not cooperate. There is not much you can do about this except to try to note that it has occurred.

During your discussions with gatekeepers, and during or immediately after your interviews, you will be taking reflexive notes of what is going on, what went wrong or went well, and how you and the task seem to be understood. You will also want to take notes of any interaction between you and your informants occurring outside the frame of the interview. These will be needed at the analysis stage and to provide reliable reflexive material for the final report.

Exercise 34: Planning an open interviewing project

Suppose you were planning an interview project to explore the nature of the health visitor's job, how would you go about it? How would you set the project up, what kinds of people would you interview, and in what way?

Summary

1 Open interviewing involves getting what people want to say, in their own words, with minimal interference of the researcher's preconceptions – though interviews may differ in the extent to which they are directive and focused on particular topics.

2 One classic form is Life-history interviewing, in which repeated interviews with a single informant (or a very small number) seek to elicit as

much detail as possible and 'surface' any possible contradictions in the informant's map of the world. This has the strengths of detail and thoroughness, but the weakness that it is restricted to one or a few informants and therefore difficult to generalize.

3 Similar methods may be used, with larger numbers, to compare groups and learn from the comparisons.

4 The purpose of such interviews is to get as close to a natural situation as can be achieved in what is patently a research situation, and this guides the manner in which the interviews are conducted.

5 The interpretation of open interview data is not simple but depends on taking a theoretical stance as to the relationship between what people say – in particular situations, in response to particular questions – and what they know, believe, feel and have experienced.

Further reading

Burgess, Robert (1984) *In the Field*. London: Allen and Unwin.
Hammersley, Martyn and Atkinson, Paul (1995) *Ethnography: Principles in Practice* (2nd edition). London: Routledge.
McCracken, Grant (1988) *The Long Interview*. Beverly Hills, CA: Sage.
Patton, Michael (1987) *How to Use Qualitative Methods in Evaluation*. Beverly Hills, CA: Sage.

Answers to Exercises

Exercise 33

Here you would be trying for a broad descriptive focus on the person's life. You would not be working towards 'treatment' at this time – except insofar as the mere act of researching a problem and taking an interest in those who suffer from it has a therapeutic effect in itself, something which has often been found. You would start by getting the informant talking about his or her childhood in general terms, probably, and lead steadily up to the present day and plans for the future. On the way through you would be taking note of anything that emerged about food, meals, poverty, attractiveness or other potentially related topics, but you would probably leave it fairly late in the series of interviews to introduce these deliberately as topics for discussion. At the end you might well find clues as to treatment for this informant or similar informants, in general. For example, using the more structured approach of the Role Repertory Grid, Fay Fransella has examined groups of obese people and also groups of stutterers, eliciting their pictures of themselves and key others in their lives, and also their picture of people who are obese or who stutter (the work is described in Bannister and Fransella 1980). The most interesting thing is that the people with the 'problem' had a quite clear picture of the kind of person who had that problem, but they did not describe themselves in those terms. It was as though, for example, the world were divided into obese people and others, and some of the 'others' (including the informant) happened to eat rather a lot.

The major drawback of the single-case life history is obviously that it *is* based on a single case. However **typical** you may suppose the informant to be, you cannot generalize from one case to a population except very tentatively. You cannot tell from the single case, for example, whether there is a single basis to obesity or whether a typology of different reasons for being obese or different roles of eating in people's lives might be more appropriate. Moreover, you do not have the power which a comparative design offers of learning from comparisons – comparing obese people with others who are not, comparing both with people who used to be obese but have lost weight, and so on. (You can do a little comparative work on the single case, however, by comparing current views with what they say about the time before they became obese – bearing in mind that the past is reconstructed here in the light of the present, and in the light of the 'demand characteristics' of the interview.)

The *strength* of the life-history approach is its sheer detail and the exhaustive nature of the interviewing. You have time, when dealing with a single case or a very small number of cases, to get as much detail as is available about everything which is of interest to you. Further, you go on interviewing till all the possible contradictions have emerged and been resolved or at least discussed, and until nothing further of use appears to be emerging ('theoretical saturation').

Exercise 34

When one of us (Abbott) undertook this kind of research, she conceptualized the purpose as 'to see how health visitors made sense of their professional role', in the light of literature which suggested that they themselves were uncertain about their role and its relationship to social work on the one hand and nursing on the other. She discussed what she intended with the Senior Lecturer in Health Studies responsible for health visiting courses in the institution where she worked as a lecturer. The Senior Lecturer gave her the names of the nurse managers in charge of health visiting in the three health districts for which training in health visiting was provided by the institution. Abbott wrote to each of these, enclosing a copy of her research proposal and asking if they would be willing to give her access to the health visitors working under them. Each of them wrote back and suggested that she went to see them; she did so, and each agreed to her request. In each district the nurse manager provided her with the names and telephone numbers of health visitors working in different settings (rural, urban, working-class or middle-class areas) and with greater or less professional experience. She contacted selected ones and explained what she wanted, and all agreed to participate.

She carried out interviews with health visitors at their place of work. Each interview lasted between 1 and 1½ hours. Beforehand, she prepared a list of topic areas she wanted to cover, to act as an *aide mémoire*, but the basic approach was life-history interviewing: she started by asking each informant why she had decided to train as a health visitor, and from this got them talking generally about their work and their professional careers. After each of the interviews she went out with each health visitor for a half or a whole day, **observing** what they did with 'cases' and talking to them further. This was to give her a greater familiarity with what health visitors actually do and an opportunity to chart their day-to-day work.

This research was very much centred on health visitors' conceptions of their own roles. If the researcher had been more interested in organizational constraints and/or official goals, she would have interviewed more senior staff. If the focus had been organization at the local level, a better approach might have been to concentrate on certain 'patches' and try to interview doctors, practice nurses, midwives, etc., as well as health visitors (and perhaps social workers – particularly if she had wanted to explore questions of the mistreatment of children). With a focus on whether health visitors deliver what their clients want, interviews with the clients themselves would have been indispensable.

ANALYSING TEXT

This chapter is concerned mostly with the analysis of qualitative data: **field notes** from **participant observation**, notes on qualitative interviews, audio tapes or secondary textual sources – diaries, newspapers, articles, historical documents and so on. All of these may be seen in some sense as 'text' – verbal material not structured for the purposes of the research as is the output of a **survey** or an **experiment**, but awaiting such structure as you can impose on it or draw out of it. Qualitative data, even more than quantitative, do not speak for themselves, however much they may appear to do so; they need to be analysed. (Text may also be analysed by quantitative methods – measuring the frequency of occurrence of a topic or a concept or a word, or the space given to it in a report, or in some other way reducing the complexity of the material to analysable numbers.) In this chapter we shall talk about the descriptive use of qualitative materials, about **holistic** analysis in terms of 'cases', and about analyses in terms of the detailed content of interviews or documents. These forms of analysis blur into each other, as we shall see, but it is useful to separate them out and consider them separately here.

The first step is to get the material into a form in which it can be ordered and analysed. Tapes need to be transcribed, for example – or if you do not have the time for this (an hour's interview takes several hours to transcribe) then you at least need to take detailed notes from the tapes, plus an index of what is where (by noting the counter reading on your tape recorder which corresponds with each topic). You will need to work out a system for locating material – perhaps case numbers or day records, page numbers within them, and line numbers within the pages – so that it is possible to locate particular references easily at a later stage. You will need to read all the material you have collected, to familiarize yourself fully with it and form a tentative overall impression of it. You need also to establish a filing system. This may be physical: storing relevant material together in one place, such as a series of clearly labelled envelopes or wallet files. In this case you will need multiple copies of all your material, as some of it may well need to be stored under a number of different headings. Alternatively, your filing system may be indexical – you may 'store' references in the form of location indicators, on file cards or on the computer. (Indexical 'storage' is easier in the early stages, involving less physical transfer of material, but physical means of storage are far less trouble when it comes time to write up, as you have your source material already segmented and organized into 'sets'. However, some computerized analysis packages – for example, NUD.IST – offer the advantages of both approaches.)

The amount of data that you will have collected may well be vast, and you may feel that it is a daunting task that faces you. The first thing to do is to focus down and remind yourself what the purpose of your inquiry was, what you were interested in finding out. You will then realize that quite a lot of the material you have collected is not relevant to this. It may be interesting in its own right, and you may want to keep it to analyse at some time in the future, but it is not needed for your immediate purposes. When we interviewed mothers whose children had learning difficulties, for example, one copy of the transcribed interviews filled six or eight box files. A relatively small amount of that was relevant to what we were originally investigating: the load on the mother as compared with mothers of 'unlabelled' children, and the social and self-stigmatizing that occurred (Abbott and Sapsford 1987b, among other reports). More detailed material from a few particularly interesting 'cases' yielded another paper, on the *diversity* of mothers' experiences (Abbott and Sapsford 1986). The rest sits in the cupboard, brought out only for teaching examples, until such time as one of us wants to use it for another purpose – perhaps some kind of analysis of socialization and growing up, as we elicited the women's life histories as well as their current circumstances.

Qualitative description

Much of your material will be descriptive – describing situations and events – and you will want to use it in writing a descriptive account in your final report. Description could be a main purpose of your research. For example, in some research on evaluating Enterprise in Higher Education (EHE) which one of us (Abbott) carried out, the report on qualitative evaluation of individual enterprise programmes requires that there be a description of the programme, including the aims and objectives of its leaders, what they did and what the outcomes were. The descriptive material may itself begin the analysis by the way it is ordered under headings – e.g. in the EHE example, the programme as a whole and individual programmes as broad headings, and relevant sub-headings within each broad category. (You will find that much of the work of qualitative analysis involves sorting into hierarchical categories, in one way or another.) Careful reading of your data and thinking about what 'story' your report is to tell will enable you to decide on relevant sub-headings. All of the material for the descriptive account can be collected together and put in a file or series of envelopes labelled 'descriptive material'.

Under some circumstances it may be relevant to work through each case or setting or visit or whatever in some detail, organizing the material under relevant sub-headings. For example, if you had life-history data on a person, you could separate the purely descriptive material from the rest and organize it chronologically and under separate headings – e.g. 'child-hood relations with parents', 'education' . . . Even where this is not a relevant way of proceeding, however, it is good practice to write brief notes telling the story of each case – summarizing in a few sentences what the informant has to say about himself or herself, his or her life and the topics which are of particular interest to you, or what the significance of the setting or programme appeared to be to you and to the participants. (This may also allow your **reflexive** notes about particular data-collection sessions to have some impact on the analysis.) You may never use these overall summary accounts in your written report, but they will help to shape your analysis, and comparing them across cases may allow interesting patterns to emerge. They are also a good early point of the analysis at which to think about the informant as a whole person. (Note, however, that a proportion of published research on medicine, psychotherapy, counselling and social work draws on this kind of impressionistic material – 'case notes' – as a prime source, treating it as factual rather than as field notes of a process of participant observation and failing to acknowledge the role of the researcher/practitioner in the construction of the data.)

Case analysis

Qualitative analysis which goes beyond description consists essentially of the processes of sorting, comparing/contrasting and consolidating. Most of what follows involves, in one way or another, sorting cases or propositions or utterances or words into categories such that the members resemble each other and differ from other categories in ways which are of interest to the researcher.

The simplest form of such analysis is 'impressionistic' case analysis, sorting cases into 'heaps' which have something in common which they do not share with other cases. This is what we did at one stage of the analysis of the interviews with mothers of children with learning difficulties. We read through the transcripts of interviews and formed impressions about the mothers who were speaking, holistically rather than on the basis of any particular detailed feature of what was said. On this basis we sorted mothers (families) into those who effectively denied that a problem existed, those who acknowledged that a problem existed and were trying to cope with it (distinguishing between those who had some expressed long-term strategy and those who appeared to be keeping their heads above water on a more day-to-day basis), and those who had managed to reconstruct the situation as one with positive advantages. This kind of analysis is faithful to the data in the sense that it draws on the interview material and uses it as a basis for classification. It is obviously also open, however, to being very strongly influenced by the researchers' previous ideas, because

there are no rigorous criteria for determining wh?
other than the impressions of the researchers.

More rigorous analysis involves more detailed
within interviews, rather than just comparison
see. Even so, however, you ought to return to ι.
cases at some point of the analysis. In writing up yʊ.
want to give more detailed accounts of a subset of cases – pʊₒ.
trate different categories or types that you have 'discovered' in
research. For example, in the EHE research the final report could include a
detailed analysis of a small number of programmes as examples illustrating
the range and the kinds of enterprise they represent. Alternatively, the
cases could be selected to illustrate successful and unsuccessful programmes or to illustrate the types of problems encountered by programme
leaders in implementing the programmes, and/or students, and/or collaborating employers. All the material relevant to each of the cases needs to be
collected together – one file or envelope per case or one index entry.

Content analysis

In your subsequent analysis and write-up of these cases you would look for
similarities and differences between them. This is the main process of
bringing order to the material, organizing it into patterns, categories and
descriptive units. It is now possible to purchase computer programs that
can assist in the content analysis of qualitative data, but most of us still
have to do some or all of it by hand. Content analysis needs to be done on
all the data, including material which you have already sorted out to use
for description or as illustrative cases.

The first step is to look for all concepts and make an index of them. A
computer qualitative analysis program will do this for you, as indeed will
some word-processing packages. Using such a program, you would need to
look at its output, eliminate the very rare concepts (after looking to see
where they occurred, in case they were important) and grouping others
together because they clearly expressed similar ideas even if different
words were used. If you have to do it by hand you need to re-read every bit
of the data, noting down all the categories that are relevant to the purpose
of your analysis – and probably some that do not seem relevant at present,
but might seem so at a later stage. First you would look across the paragraphs to see what overall topic areas came up – work, home, geographical
area and its significance, the children and so on. Each of these may want
breaking down further: children's health, the children's school as a place,
the children's school performance as a measure of their worth, sports activities and so on. Finally, you might still want or need to do a full textual
analysis, looking for every descriptive category the informant uses (in
which case you might seriously consider whether you can get hold of computer assistance).

As a brief example of this kind of content analysis, consider the following
short extract from one of our interviews with a mother whose child had
learning difficulties:

RJS: What was Wyvern like when you first came here?

Mrs Weaver: It's built up a lot since we first came here. It used to be very, very quiet, very quiet.

RJS: Did you have this house then?

Mrs Weaver: No we lived in Dunstone Estate when we first moved here . . . and then we moved up here. A very friendly place, I think, Wyvern . . . It's nice. And everybody's accepted Carl [mentally handicapped son], that's what we like. In a normal way.

In this brief extract we can see a number of 'place' references qualified by adjectives – 'quiet' (as a term of approval), 'friendly', 'nice'. The topic of the mentally handicapped son has also come up, leading to concepts of 'accepting' (by people around) and 'in a *normal* way'. Another person might characterize the same place as 'quiet' (in a pejorative sense), 'nosy', 'dull'. Contrasting people who look at it in the one light or the other, we might find other differences between them – in demographic characteristics, or in the way they see their mentally handicapped children as fitting into the life of the area – and we would be on the way towards model-building. Analysis proceeds by constantly comparing and contrasting interview scripts, looking for similarities and differences, and trying to find which characteristics seem to vary systematically together.

Note that there are two levels at which this kind of analysis can be carried out. On the one hand, you can categorize the material in terms of your own previous interests. In the EHE example, for instance, the categories which are likely to emerge are very likely to be conditioned by the focus of the research. If your enquiry had a wider and less directed focus – e.g. 'What is it like being a prisoner, or a patient or a mother' – then you would want to start further back, by trying to list *all* the descriptive nouns, adjectives and phrases that look even vaguely relevant to the enquiry, clustering them by similarity, and looking further at ones that are at all common or appear to express strong feeling, *before* focusing on particular questions that may be of concern to the researcher. Except where the focus of the research is very narrow and/or the interviews were very directive, the latter is probably a better procedure than the former.

When you have a list of categories you can group them into sets of similar relevance and begin to map their relationships. For example, in our research into community care for children with special learning difficulties we grouped all the concepts relating to 'husband', 'children', 'mother', 'other kin', the ones relating to 'neighbours', to 'schools' and so on. These were clusters which appeared to make sense to the informants and which made sense to us. There is no magic formula for how concepts are to be clustered – you are just looking for ones that appear to go together, express the same underlying idea or are related to the same topic sub-area. The clusters can again be grouped more broadly in further analysis – 'husband' and 'children' go together as 'nuclear family', 'mother' and 'other kin' go together as 'kin network'. At this stage, as far as is possible, the themes and categories should come from the data rather than from previous ideas – they should reflect patterns found more than patterns looked for.

Meta-analysis

The aim so far has been to try to characterize the informants' worlds in the terms in which they themselves see them. The next step – what one might call 'second-order analysis' – is to go beyond the informants' concepts and start trying to build theory at another level. Patterns may suggest themselves in the data. For example, the people who saw places such as Wyvern as 'nice' may tend to be those with mentally handicapped children of school age or preschool children who were not handicapped; those who saw it as 'dull' might have older children, or very young children who were handicapped. We hasten to say that this is *not* the pattern we found in our interview study. If it *had* occurred, however, we might have speculated about the different needs of the four types of families, for activities for themselves and the children, and started building a model of the school-age mentally handicapped child as having some of the social function of the preschool non-handicapped child (i.e. constituting the same kind of burden). We might look for further confirmation in what informants did *not* say. Might it be the case, for example, that those who found Wyvern dull talked about a need for entertainment or relaxation, while those who found it 'nice' did not? Was this a difference which held up across time – were the latter less likely to mention entertainment and relaxation even when talking about their lives before marriage? Or might it be an adaptation to circumstances: did the latter fail to mention relatives or friends able to look after the child while they went out? Or might it be the perception of the former which was at fault: perhaps they lacked a support network and, therefore, felt confined, while the latter were, in fact, able to get out when they wanted to? All of this is going substantially beyond what any one informant might want to say about his or her life, but it is still analysis grounded in data, and the informants might still recognize themselves in this account.

This is a particular example of a general principle – looking for how respondents typify or stereotype or categorize the field of the research, and drawing generalized conclusions from the patterns that emerge. In the example above we were looking at judgements of place, but it might have been judgements they make and express about other people, or government agencies, or medical procedures, depending on the topic area of the research. For example, research on nurses has shown them typifying patients into 'good' and 'bad' categories, and the category within which a patient was placed has an effect on the ways in which the nurses treated and interacted with him or her. In our research on mothers, they typified health visitors as 'helpful' and 'unhelpful', and separately into 'informed', 'ignorant' and 'bossy' ('ignorant, but not prepared to admit it'). Relatives were categorized as 'helpful', 'unhelpful' or 'indifferent'. The categories were not necessarily related; a health visitor could be ignorant, but helpful. Sometimes a typificatory scheme will be used by all respondents. Sometimes it will be used by some, with others using a different one; in the research above, for example, some mothers regarded *all* health visitors (and, we thought, all *conceivable* health visitors) as 'unhelpful'. Sometimes it will be unique to a particular informant. Once the typologies have been identified and the relevant material sorted out, it is possible to start asking serious questions about the content: what is it that is seen as making 'a good patient', 'a helpful health visitor', 'an indifferent relative'?

Exercise 35: Analysis of interview data

Try your hand at some analysis, with the following brief extract from one of our interviews with mothers of children with learning disabilities. Our initial shot at it is given at the end of the chapter. (All names are fictitious. The phrases in square brackets are our interpolations.)

RJS: You think Kings School [ESN(S) school for children with severe learning disabilities] has been bringing him on?

Mrs Weaver: Oh yeah, marvellous, yeah! He's only been there 12 months, and we've noticed a vast, er, change in him . . . it was me, I pushed, I didn't want him to go to Kings because I'd heard so much of, I'm a bit frightened of that sort of thing, I, I don't like illness, you know?

RJS: Hm.

Mrs Weaver: And I'd heard so much about all the terrible sort of cases there . . . But [the ESN(M) school for children with mild learning disabilities] wasn't really the sort of place for him. It's for maladjusted rather than handicapped children, you know. And I mean, they did all they could for him, but the last 12, 18 months he was there he was ever so miserable . . . they're very good at Kings, you know. I mean, if there's any problems they're straight away, sort of, on to you, telling you. They involve you in everything. And as I say, he's happy there.

RJS: Does he get, does he get on with the other children?

Mrs Weaver: Yeah, yeah, he does, everyone seems to like him. But Carl's like that, he's got a way with him, everybody sort of takes to him . . .

PAA: What, he went to a, to a nursery, did he, at [the ESN(M) school]?

Mrs Weaver: Yes, he started when he was, I think he was, I can't really remember how old he was, he must have been about three, and he went there until last year, as I say.

PAA: Then he was assessed as educable?

Mrs Weaver: Oh, yeah . . . The last time he was assessed there, it was Mr Bowen, the what do you call it?

PAA: Psychologist.

Mrs Weaver: Yeah, that's right. He said 'Oh, he's not yet reached the mental age of a two-year-old', and I was most insulted, you know. I mean, I know he has, I mean, a two-year-old didn't do what Carl was doing.

RJS: Yes

Mrs Weaver: Um, and I think it's unfair that they assess them like they do. I mean he, he took Carl into a room, and Carl had

> never seen him before, and he wouldn't do anything for
> him, and he kept saying 'He doesn't know where his nose
> is, doesn't know where this, that and the other is', and I
> felt like saying, 'Well, you get him in here, and I'll show
> you whether he knows where it is', you know.
> RJS: Yes [*laughs*]
> Mrs Weaver: I mean, he'd not even seen the man before. Carl was very
> afraid of strangers then . . . But this psychologist, I mean I
> don't really think he gave him the benefit of the doubt
> then. I mean, I knew that Carl knew them things, but I'm
> not the sort of person to say 'Well, I know that he knows
> that', you know.

A final stage in the analysis is to go beyond the patterns that are emergent in the data themselves and try to *explain* them – a theoretical interpretation. In our research on the mothers, for example, we typified them on the basis of our analysis of the material we had collected. We also put their experiences into the context of policies of community care and examined the extent to which our findings matched those of other researchers. Furthermore, we tried to locate them (in the first half of the book, which you were not directed to read) within a set of historical processes which makes sense at the same time of their reactions to their own circumstances, the reactions of others to the visibly handicapped children, and the nature and development of government policy in this area.

However far you go along the road of analysis, meta-analysis and theoretical interpretation – even if you do not get far beyond 'description' – it is important to 'test' tentative conclusions by looking back through the material for contradictory evidence – for material that will challenge or question the interpretation you have put on your findings. It is also important to be continually reflexive – to consider how your purpose, your training, your reading, your background assumptions and your prejudices have influenced both the collection of the data and your analysis of them. It can be useful to write notes relevant to this as you are doing the analysis, and it is certainly wise to try to keep a log or diary of the stages of the analysis. These themselves become data for analysis. A good starting point is to write down all your initial ideas, past findings, hopes for the research, ideas about what you think you might find, at the outset of the research, and continue to make notes as you go along.

Ideology and discourse

Working with textual material as text, some research will call for a leap straight into a form of meta-analysis. Sometimes the interest focuses not on the detailed content, but on what is expressed by it – **ideologies, discourses**, settled 'world-views' which emerge from the way that topics are discussed. This is sometimes called **critical analysis**. It has most often been applied in the analysis of government documents and the utterances of politicians, particularly in the criminological field, looking for politically informed views of the world that are implicit in what is being said and taken for granted, unanalysed, by the speaker or writer. Similar work has been done by feminists on texts about education, family and social policy. Such work is necessarily impressionistic, but what emerges can be very illuminating.

Critical analysis often goes beyond both the text and the ideologies or models which it expresses to apply a 'sociology of knowledge' perspective to the text and look at the circumstances of its production. If we treat a text not as just a declaration of an author's views but a response to a situation, located within a history of both texts and practices and responding to a history of attacks and resistance, we can often achieve a different kind or level of understanding of it. A government minister's speech on health policy and finance, for example, is not just an expression of his or her views and intentions, nor is it just to be read for the political and domestic ideologies that it embodies – though these will often be very illuminating! It also has a place in the history of that government's policy – a continuation, a redirection or, possibly, a redirection masquerading under the banner of continuity. It will be more extreme than anything previous, or represent a turning away from an unpopularly extreme position, or continue and reinforce some current policy (and therefore defensive, if the policy is unpopular, or 'cashing in' on the policy's popularity). It will represent a greater involvement of government or a greater shift of responsibility (with or without resources) to the domestic or commercial spheres. Finally, it will reflect the popularity of the Party, the popularity of its policies and, probably, the time remaining to the next general election. All of these factors help to shape it, and we can understand it better by putting it in this kind of context.

Discourse analysis is a similar development which has become very influential during the last ten years in sociology, social psychology and feminist research. It works from the same premises as critical analysis in that it tends to regard texts not as productions of people but as expressions of dominant or subversive *ideologies* or *discourses*. (We shall define these two terms below, but you should note that the definitions will be too simple. They are both ideas which can be apprehended and used at a simple level – they are not complex in essence – but they have been much elaborated by philosophical sociologists and psychologists and constitute a battleground for philosophical positions too abstruse, though important, to be considered here.)

For our purposes here we may define an *ideology* as a (superficially) coherent collection of ideas and beliefs, masquerading as 'knowledge', which purport to characterize some part of the social and natural world, express the truth about it and declare how one ought to behave with respect to it. They will give the impression that this behaviour is in the interests of some subordinate group, but the ideas will also (or instead!) serve the interests of a dominant group. One example would be the cluster of ideas around men as in competition, the need for men to work, the dignity of labour, the naturalness of receiving wages in proportion to time spent working, the rightness of the market as a mechanism for fixing those wages, the immorality of idleness and profligacy, the degrading nature of 'charity', the need to demonstrate one's respectability by job position and to augment it by 'climbing the social ladder', and so on. There is nothing *wrong* with these ideas, and we adhere to many of them, but they are a product of our culture and history (not shared by many other cultures) and are curiously consonant with the needs of a capitalist mode of production. Another example would be the cluster of ideas around the natural ability of women to care and tend, their preference for cooperation, their natural altruism, the rightness of a domestic division of labour with men as bread-winners and women as home-makers, the greater right of men than women to paid employment, women's need for community respect, the production and rearing of children as something by which women can rea-sonably be judged, the need of children for the continuous presence of a female biological parent, the importance of children's needs coming first, and so on. Again some of these ideas may be reasonable, though some of them express 'truths' of biology which are factually false, but the most notable things about them is that as a 'package' they are less than 200 years old and that they favour men over women to a very marked extent.

If an ideology is a set of propositions (or practices capable of being expressed propositionally) which declare what the truth is about the world, a *discourse* is the framework or language within which such propos-itions are set. A discourse does not declare a proposition true or false, but it sets (a) the rules by which truth or falsity is to be judged, and (b) the way that objects are to be defined and identified. A dominant 'rule of truth' in current discourses is the scientific one of appeal to conclusions based on openly available evidence, and this is what we tend to call up immediately when asked to talk about truth or falsity. Other rules are both possible and used, however: authority (not 'here is the evidence', but 'the scientists say' or 'the experts say', tradition ('it's always been done this way', 'I learned as a child that this is the right way to do things') and, indeed, morality/ aesthetics ('whatever the outcome, this is the proper way to behave and the right way to live your life'). The definition of 'objects' is a more subtle fea-ture of discourses but possibly even more important. Consider, for example, the discourses within which domestic ideology is set and their use of the terms 'family', 'home', 'wife', 'mother', 'husband', 'child'. These make possible sentences such as 'For the sake of the family it is best that wives build the home while their husbands provide resources, and a mother's first duty is to her child, not her own career.' Translating this into a different discourse we might get 'For the sake of those who live together in the same house and are related biologically or by marriage, it is best that females undertake domestic labour while co-resident males undertake industrial labour for pay which they share with the females, and a female worker (but not a male one) should put the interests of any offspring they might have above those of her own employment.' Somehow the second sentence does not have the same inherent plausibility as the first! (Gender itself may be seen as a discursive device: to bring gender into a discussion is to assert, without proof or, often, evidence, that there is some inherent dif-ference between males and females.)

Some discourse analysis is critical analysis, looking at relations of power: how underlying ideologies and their supporting discourses have developed over time and interacted with social institutions in the interests of some groups over others. Notable here is the work of Michel Foucault (1963, 1975, 1976) on the reform of criminals, the growth of modern medicine and the nature of sexuality, and subsequent work by Nikolas Rose (1985, 1989) and Wendy Hollway (1991). Another approach, however, looks not at discursive forms and their history but at how discourses are *used* in practice to establish dominance, to legitimate knowledge and to control the behaviour and even the minds of others. Here notable examples would be the work of Jonathan Potter and Margaret Wetherell (Potter and Wetherell 1987; Wetherell and Potter 1992; Wetherell 1995) on gender identity and on racism, and Michael Billig's *et al.*'s (1988) work on racism and on power relations between different grades of staff in medicine.

Summary

1 Analysing text is largely a matter of indexing the segments of the material and arranging them in categories to 'make sense of them' or 'tell a meaningful tale'. *What* tale is to be told will be a matter of what the researcher wants to get out of the research.

2 At the lowest level, there is a role for simply trying to 'tell the story' (provide a précis) of each interview or case – to get across what the informant was trying to get across, succinctly and with irrelevancies and diversions left out.

3 The next level of analysis involves the comparison and contrast of cases – looking for similarities and differences, and sorting cases into categories on dimensions which appear to be of importance to the informants or to you as researcher.

4 At one remove further from just expressing what the informants have to say comes content analysis – the detailed analysis of the concepts used by informants and their interrelation. Content analysis tries to put together an overall description or model of the way in which the informant sees the world (with reference, probably, to a specific topic area which is your research interest). This model may or may not be recognizable to the informants, in the sense that it may or may not present a way of categorizing their lives which they already employ.

5 At the next level comes what we have termed 'meta-analysis', which is quite definitely concerned with making sense *to the researcher* rather than the informant; it employs the researcher's theoretical categories rather than the everyday ones familiar to the informant.

6 At the extreme of meta-analysis lies critical analysis or discourse analysis, which is concerned not with the meaning of what the informant has to say but with the ideologies or discourses which inform what is said and of which the text is 'symptomatic', and with the social and historical context within which the text is produced.

Further reading

Burgess, Robert (1984) *In the Field*. London: Allen and Unwin.

Hammersley, Martyn and Atkinson, Paul (1995) *Ethnography: Principles in Practice* (2nd edition). London: Routledge.

Hyener, R.H. (1985) Some guidelines for the phenomenological analysis of interview data, *Human Problems*, 8: 279–303.

Jupp, Victor (1993) Critical analysis of text, Unit 21 of Open University course DEH313, *Principles of Social and Educational Research*.

Patton, Michael (1987) *How to Use Qualitative Methods in Evaluation*. Beverly Hills, CA: Sage.

Plummer, Kenneth (1983) *Documents of Life*. London: Allen and Unwin.

Potter, Jonathan and Wetherell, Margaret (1987) *Discourse and Social Psychology: Beyond Attitudes and Behaviour*. London: Sage.

Smith, Jonathan, Harre, Rom and Van Langenhove, Luk (1995) *Rethinking Methods in Social Psychology*. London: Sage (Chapter 6).

Specimen answer to Exercise 35

The overall story is a clear one, of assessment by an educational psychologist whom Mrs Weaver sees as incompetent, testing her child under conditions where Carl could not possibly do his best. This is what she was telling us in this passage. It is not clear from what is here whether this is seen as a failure of this particular psychologist or as characteristic of the breed. The passage is a brief one, but descriptive categories do emerge which would be worth following up through the rest of the script and other scripts:

1 Describing herself, Mrs Weaver talks about herself with negative emotion as 'pushing' on a particular occasion and as 'frightened of that sort of thing' [severely disabled cases in the ESN(S) school], and in positive terms as 'not the sort of person' to push her views forward. Carl, positively, is described as 'everyone seems to like him . . . he's got a way with him'. 'Afraid of strangers', applied to Carl, does not seem to be a negative label so much as a neutral description of a childhood stage. This begins to give us a basis for understanding her ways of categorizing other people, which could be followed up in the rest of the interview and contrasted with other interviews.

2 The description of the assessment process is interestingly juridical, in the use of the phrase 'didn't give him the benefit of the doubt' and in the repeated description of it as 'unfair'.

3 We should note that, like any other parent, Mrs Weaver's honour is bound up in the outcome of the test: 'He said, "Oh, he's not yet reached the mental age of a two-year-old", and I was most insulted.'

4 The terms used to describe children who have been classified as mentally handicapped are interesting: 'that sort of thing, I don't like illness', 'terrible sort of cases there', 'maladjusted' (of the 'mild' children), 'handicapped' of her own (without the qualifying 'mentally').

5 What is missing, from this passage and, in fact, from the whole interview, is any use of phrases such as 'these children' to refer to mentally
handicapped children as a class. Mrs Weaver does not show the signs evident in some of the interviews of classing them together as something
different from herself. On the contrary, the force of her early remarks
about fears of Kings School on the one hand, and the description of children in the other school as not really handicapped, is to separate him
from both and render him unique.

PARTICIPANT OBSERVATION

In this chapter we look at the broadest, most **naturalistic** and least pre-structured form of research: observing in a natural setting, as a participant. This is one way in which situations have been explored from the perspective of the participants with (ideally) minimal imposition of researchers' or managements' preconceived ideas. It is also one form in which your own practice may be investigated in the widest possible way, looking not at how some particular practice works, but at how, in general, your professional life is lived, what it means and what the implicit 'working rules' are.

Deliberately, we have not set practical exercises in this chapter. **Participant observation** might be seen as the most dangerous way in which research can be conducted. It can be destructive of relationships, it can upset and sidetrack your professional practice, and the 'methodological imagination' can sometimes be stretched to the point where your very sense of identity comes under attack. You can also do great damage to the people in the context you are researching, if the practice of your research is not constantly monitored by you and by others. It is not a form of research to be undertaken without supervision from someone who has been 'in the field' and knows the problems, and from an academic base where, at frequent intervals, you can change roles and discharge the tensions and self-doubts which have accumulated during the fieldwork.

Covert participant observation

In this section we shall talk about classic participant observation, where a researcher becomes part of a context without participants knowing that he or she is a researcher – **covert** (hidden, secret) participant observation. A first and substantial problem, clearly, is how the researcher is to become part of the context. Sometimes it is possible to join by legitimate means: one may do participant observation in a hospital by coming in legitimately as a patient, for example, or by becoming a student nurse, or by taking a job as a hospital porter, or by joining the 'Friends of the Hospital' and acquiring the role of the person who takes a trolley of books round or the person who works in the hospital shop. If you wanted to do research on childcare and you had children, it would be easy enough to *join* the relevant playgroup or parent–teacher association or to place your children with childminders and take notes of what goes on. In many contexts it is not possible to join in this way, however. If you wanted to do research on student doctors, for example, it might not be possible for you to join as a medical student. It might be possible, however, for you to pass yourself off as a student doctor – to dress similarly and to attend the same lectures and demonstrations. Research on youths, on unemployed persons, on 'deviant' sexual groups and on religious sects has been carried out by this stratagem of *passing* – pretending to be a relevant person within the context.

A second problem is data collection, because quite clearly any sign that you were taking notes as you went along would destroy your credibility as a genuine participant. Sometimes it is possible to take notes in a covert manner, but within the normal actions of a participant – if paperwork is normally conducted, or if one can seem to be reading something and scribbling in the margins. More often it is necessary to leave the scene from time to time to take notes (going to the toilet, for example – the first sign of a covert participant observer is often an apparently weak bladder!), or 'writing up' at the end of a session or the end of the day. Whatever stratagem has to be adopted, it is crucial to make as full a record as possible, as soon as possible, before events and occurrences have begun to be rearranged in memory.

The full-blown participant enquiry is not just an intuitive description. At first one goes into the field in a descriptive way, establishes a role, learns the part and just tries to get a feel for what is going on. As the observation progresses, however, ideas will begin to emerge as to what it is important to say about the context, and progressively one will begin to pay more attention to some features of the situation than to others. This *progressive focusing* is the first stage of theory-building – trying to establish what is important or interesting in the situation. As time goes on the theme will become clearer and a tentative theoretical model of the situation will begin to be put forward. This will be refined and tested by:

1 **Theoretical sampling**: testing the generality and the boundaries of an idea. One might look initially for very similar situations or aspects of a single situation, to show that the model had some generality. Next one might look for very dissimilar contexts, to establish the boundaries of the ideas. Finally, one might systematically sample groups who were like the original one in every respect but one, to test particular hypotheses. For example, working in a hospital on nurses, you would check that your emerging ideas held for the night shift as well as for the day nurses, for all types of wards, for auxiliaries, aids and students, as well as for qualified nurses. You might then try to see whether they held for sisters, for doctors, for the hospital management or whether they were confined to the 'shop floor' of the caring staff, and you might look at patients and their relatives to see whether they were applicable beyond the caring staff. Finally, you might start making very specific comparisons – male nurses

and female ones, older nurses and younger ones, theatre nurses and ward nurses – according to what your emerging model predicted might be of interest.

2 *Analytic induction*: given a model which seems to be well delineated after this kind of process, a final stage is to test it against 'unlikely cases'. You deliberately look for cases which falsify your picture or do not seem to fit the model, and to the extent that they cannot be 'explained away' you try to reformulate the model to take account of them. This process goes on until you are very sure of the boundaries of what you want to say and no new information appears to be emerging – the point of *theoretical saturation*.

(We should perhaps point out that very few projects get as far as this; what we are describing is an ideal and complete project, probably representing several years' work.)

A problem with all participant work, but particularly acute in covert participant observation, is the marginal nature of the researcher. Marginality is essential, so that the natural situation shall not be changed by the researcher's presence and so that he or she can stand back from the taken-for-granted nature of the situation. The researcher must be able to see it in a more complete and analytic way even than the participants. Marginality is very difficult to maintain, however. If the researcher remains uninvolved in the situation, the value of being a participant is lost. (It is also a very lonely and disorienting experience.) If he or she 'goes native' and becomes a true participant to the extent that the researcher's detachment is lost, then the research suffers. Finding a place between these two extremes which is effective and comfortable is very difficult. Wherever the researcher is located, short of going completely native, anxiety and stress will follow, as the researcher tries to balance the two roles while 'maintaining cover', concealing the research role and acting plausibly as what he or she purports to be in the situation.

Covert participant observation incurs further costs, in personal and ethical terms. To the extent that the researcher manages to maintain cover, he or she may be drawn into disturbing the situation by the very role that is being played: researchers have found themselves almost becoming gang leaders, for instance, because they know more about the police than the average youth and their advice is therefore good. They may also find themselves dragged into behaviour which is normal for participants (and they will 'blow their cover' if they abstain), but which they may not wish to undertake. People researching in shops and offices have had to condone pilfering, for example, or been invited to take part, and research on youth may drag the researcher into vandalism or violence. At the other extreme, if the researcher fails to maintain cover, he or she will be exposed as a fraud who had been building up relationships for the sake of research; at the least this will hurt, dismay or anger the true participants, and they may take steps against him or her as a consequence. Perhaps the worst problem, however, is how to live with the experience of building relationships and enjoying confidences with the intention of using them for a purpose unknown by the participants. The researcher may be able to cope with this if the consequences of the research are seen as important (research into commercial malpractice and the 'crimes of the powerful', for instance) or if the research is seen as putting the participants' point of view to the world, but it remains, nonetheless, an uncomfortable position. Many social scientists would now argue that covert participant observation is always ethically unacceptable.

Exercise 36: Advantages and disadvantages of *overt* observation

Spend a few minutes thinking about observation in which the researcher's identity as researcher is not concealed. What advantages do you see, and what would be the disadvantages, as compared with covert participant observation?

Overt observation

Much participant research is carried out quite openly, with the researcher being readily identifiable as a researcher. (See, for example, the Kirkham paper which we looked at in Chapter 4.) Declaring what you are saves many of the ethical qualms of covert work – no one is deceived and participants know that you cannot necessarily be expected to 'go along with' everything that they do. You also have a freedom to 'move around in the field' which is often denied the covert observer. For example, one group of covert observers had themselves admitted as patients to a mental hospital (Caudill *et al.* 1952), and learned a great deal about how patients are treated and how they treat each other. Being labelled as patients, however, they could not also observe the nurses or the doctors on their own ground and socialize with them as equals. If they had been openly researching, it would have been quite natural for them (indeed, probably required of them), to talk to people at all levels and to make themselves available in a wide range of circumstances. You are also freer to ask questions. As the 'amiable incompetent' in a covert role you can pretend to be a little stupid or ignorant in order to elicit material, but the extent to which you can do so without 'blowing your cover' is strictly limited. As a researcher no one necessarily expects you to understand what is going on, so you are free to ask.

The disadvantage is the risk of **reactivity**: that your presence and the way you behave is altering the situation and that things would be quite different if you were not there. This is a risk even in covert work – by taking a role you necessarily affect the situation. In overt work you have to make substantial allowances for the fact that people know they are being researched – something akin to a Hawthorne Effect – and for the fact that they are undoubtedly trying to 'sell you a line' of one sort or another. As time goes on and people become used to your presence you may feel that this tendency is diminishing, but you can never be sure. You may also not necessarily feel that all the ethical problems of covert work are overcome; it is still the case that you are building relationships for your own particular purposes, to gain data rather than just to relate.

Another problem even with 'open' participant research is encountered where any kind of power relationship is involved – where the setting in which the research is being carried out involves clients or patients or pupils or inmates. Not infrequently when researchers say that they were open participants in a setting they mean that their identity was known to the professionals in it – the doctors, nurses, social workers, health visitors, teachers, prison staff. Rather less often is their presence as researchers explained or even made obvious to the patients, clients, pupils or inmates. Intimate or private aspects of clients' or pupils' lives may be reported in research which did not ask for their consent to this. It is not entirely clear, in all situations, whether asking consent would be in the patients' interests: it could distort the relationship with the professionals and interfere with the effectiveness of the service they require, if they were aware that they were under research scrutiny. However, whether participant research is ethical under such circumstances must therefore be a matter for debate. Furthermore, even where consent is given by clients or pupils or patients, it is not clear how free that consent is: where someone requires a service from a professional (as in health care) or is under a professional's authority (as in schools), it is difficult to refuse such requests.

Another problem (which applies to 'open' interviewing as well) is that the informants may not have realized the 'rules of the game' as seen by the researcher. In interviews, the informant is well aware that what is said to the tape recorder will be used for the research. He or she may not be aware that what is said 'off-stage' during coffee breaks or casual meetings will also be used. (The researcher may agree not to use material which is declared to be 'not for the tape recorder', but there is no way that he or she can *avoid* using it; it is *there*, in the researcher's mind, during the analysis, and it must necessarily shape how the formally recorded material is interpreted.) Similarly, a teacher may quite happily allow a researcher to participate in classroom sessions. He or she may not feel, however, that the contract stretches to the (inevitable) use of remarks and conversations overheard in the staffroom or even the toilets.

The overarching methodological problem with reports based on participant observation data, whether covert or overt, is the problem of **validity**: why anyone should take your word that what you claim to have seen and heard is what any other reasonable person would have extracted from the situation. Inevitably, however much you illustrate your report with quotations and extracts from field notes, the reader has to trust you to have interpreted what you saw, heard and experienced in the same way that he or she would have interpreted it. The two guarantors of validity to which you may make appeal are **triangulation** and **reflexivity**. Triangulation, a metaphor drawn from navigation, means taking more than one bearing on a point in order to locate it uniquely. In research terms it means being able to show that more than one source has been used, each with its own bias, but not necessarily the same in each case. Thus observation is supplemented with interviews, to show that what you conclude from observing behaviour is what the participants also understand by it, or at least that what you conclude makes sense to the participants. One may draw on informal conversations overheard in staffrooms, toilets, etc. to supplement formal interviews. One may look for diaries, letters, articles which participants have written for the newspapers, etc. in order to extend the range of perspectives. Ideally, one may have more than one observer, perhaps located in different parts of the 'research field', to elicit different viewpoints and different interpretations. Each of these sources leads to an account, and no account is necessarily privileged over other accounts, but to the extent that differently based accounts appear to agree we may have more faith in the result. To the extent that they do not agree, further research may be needed before you are in a position to report.

Reflexivity is of even more importance. At every stage of the research, right from the initial introductions, you must be thinking about how the participants are making sense of you and your presence, what you are taking for granted or learning as new about them, and how what you are doing may be shaping particular pieces of data or the whole relationship between you and participants. This is important for three reasons. It acts as a form of self-monitoring, so that you can spot something going wrong and be at pains to correct it. It is, itself, a form of data analysis, one way in which you find your way through the morass of material towards the underlying model which simplifies and makes sense of what is going on. Finally, it is the basis of your self-justification in the eventual report, your way of showing that others should believe that your interpretations are reasonable ones.

Observation in the workplace

There are obvious advantages in being a 'participant observer' in your own workplace, but equally obvious disadvantages, given what we have said above. The major advantage is that you already have a natural role, the one you are carrying out in your job. There is no question of 'joining' or 'passing': you are already *in*. Equally important, at a practical level, you have no need to find your way through a maze of 'gatekeepers': you are already in the situation and can take whatever notes it pleases you to take with no need for anyone's permission. (You may find your superiors feel they should have been consulted if you ever decide to publish anything from your notes, but if what is at stake is a piece of 'internal research', examining and drawing conclusions from the practice and ethos of your unit, then no one can restrain you from doing it.) The overwhelming problem, however, is that you are a part of what you are examining. It is very difficult indeed to stand back from your normal practices and see them as anything other than the only or best way of coping with the situation. It is very difficult to stand back from the normal assumptions and typifications of your trade, and see them as anything other than inevitable and sensible. (Sensible they may be, but it is a necessary part of taking the research stance that you do not regard them as inevitable but try to see them as what *happens* to be there, among the wide range of what *might* have been there.) All this may require you to put aside your own values and goals and your professional socialization; you work in a situation you may have struggled for years to make familiar, but the research requires that you stand back from it and make it strange to yourself. Most difficult of all is to put down your own automatic assumptions about what is normal, sensible, right in any given situation and ask yourself, first, whether others hold the same values and, secondly, whether what you all do may also (or instead) serve some other purpose.

A good starting-point for such research is autobiography. Spend a good period of time trying to describe your own life and values on paper, from before you ever joined the given line of work to the present day, covering what you think the job is for, what you want out of it (not necessarily the same question), where you would like to go next, what you think brings others into the job, what you think motivates them, whether it motivates you. Study this record as if it were a set of life-history interviews conducted with someone else, and analyse it for major themes; learn from these themes what your own preconceptions are likely to be. Better still – because diary-writing of this kind is still shaped by the presence of an 'other in the head', an other who looks for socially acceptable positions – get someone else to interview you and ask the questions; others can push you to clarify ideas which might seem to you self-evidently clear when you write them down. Best of all, do both – but write the autobiography before undergoing the interview, because both are fallible accounts and the power of an interviewer to make you clarify what you might otherwise have passed over is likely to affect any subsequent account that you write.

Whether working covertly or overtly, you have to be very careful about your working relationships when researching your own work setting. A clear distinction must be made here between 'research' – activities leading to a publication or a report to management or even a set of conclusions announced in public – and the monitoring of your own daily practice, and the practice of staff for whom you are responsible, which is a necessary part of most professional jobs and can benefit from the application of research techniques and the research imagination. Monitoring must be done and, therefore, should be done well. 'Research' is something undertaken additionally, and faces the ethical problems of participant research which have been discussed earlier in the chapter – problems of interfering in the working lives of colleagues and clients/patients, with or without their consent. You will necessarily find yourself asking questions which probe into a level of intimacy which may not be appropriate for the stage of acquaintanceship which you have reached. Even if you do not find people 'cooling' to your inquisitiveness, you will find yourself in possession of information which would normally be appropriate to a much closer level of intimacy than you have so far reached, because you will have paid attention to people in a way that you would not normally as part of your everyday working life. Handling this at the personal level can be a problem. In open research – or even more, in covert research when your cover is blown and people realize that you are taking notes on them – you can become labelled as a spy or a reporter, someone with whom interaction has to be very guarded.

Perhaps more difficult still is the effect of researching your own working milieu and its 'normal rules' on your relationship to your own professional practice. Our professional lives depend in large part on the values which we have incorporated, and on a set of working practices and priorities which have become largely unconscious by the time that we have become competent at our trades. To stand back and question these can be like the priest questioning his faith and his commitment to the church – once we 'make the familiar strange', it may *remain* strange, and we may not be able to find our way back to professional commitment. The methodological imagination involves a great degree of self-questioning, and those (which is most of us) who are unsure of themselves should be careful how deeply they question something as crucial to their public and private identities as their professional roles and practices.

A way round some of these problems is the **collaborative** approach. If a whole group of you get together to assess and evaluate how you do your job together, then the loneliness is dispelled, you are not faced with taking the role of the spy, and there are others with whom you can talk out personal problems that may arise in the course of the research. Three warnings, however:

1 There is no 'natural situation' for you to explore: what you have is the contrived situation of a group of people who are all committed to a programme of research and improvement, and who are all watching themselves and each other. The 'autobiography' stage, or prior interviewing of each other, is particularly important here.
2 A Hawthorne Effect, or something akin, is inevitable: what you will be exploring is not normal practice, but how practice can be improved by and during collaborative evaluation.
3 Once started, such an undertaking is difficult to stop, and the atmosphere of the unit can become very intense and critical.

Summary

1 Participant observation may be *overt* or *covert*. In the latter the researcher takes a position in the field and conceals the fact that research is going on. In the former he or she is a declared researcher but still tries to become a part of the natural life which is being observed.

2 The major advantage of covert observation is its naturalism – it disturbs the context as little as possible. It is not always easy to find a plausible role, however; there is always the danger of 'breaking cover', and data collection may be physically difficult to arrange if it is to remain concealed. There are also substantial ethical problems in invading people's lives without their knowledge or permission.

3 Overt observation avoids these problems, and it is easier for the researcher to 'move around the field' and vary methods, thereby obtaining greater coverage. However, the known presence of the researcher must have some distorting effect.

4 Observation research is not just intuitive description. The researcher builds models of what is going on and what it means to participants, and tests them through **theoretical sampling**.

5 Reflexivity is extremely important in all observation research. The researcher must be alive to all possible reactive effects, including how he

or she is received by the participants and what the nature of the research (if overt) is considered to be.

6 The observer needs to be able to 'make the familiar strange'. That is, he or she must be enough immersed in the situation and its meanings to understand it at least to some extent in the same way as the participants understand it, but sufficiently detached not to take for granted what the participants take for granted.

7 This is a particularly difficult stance to maintain when trying to carry out observation research in a setting where one is a natural participant, because one already has a role in the situation and a stake in the outcomes.

8 There are again substantial problems – both personal and ethical – with carrying out research into a context which forms part of your own life. There is great danger of violating trust, and your own relationships and taken-for-granted participation may be disturbed or fragmented.

Further reading

Burgess, Robert (1984) *In the Field*. London: Allen and Unwin.

Hammersley, Martyn and Atkinson, Paul (1995) *Ethnography: Principles in Practice* (2nd edition). London: Routledge.

Patton, Michael (1987) *How to Use Qualitative Methods in Evaluation*. Beverly Hills, CA: Sage.

Taylor, S.J. and Bogden, R. (1984) *An Introduction to Qualitative Research Methods*. Chichester: Wiley.

For a straightforward account of a piece of participant work, see:

Cavendish, Ruth (1982) *Women on the Line*. London: Routledge and Kegan Paul.

IN CONCLUSION

WRITING UP

When the research is finished, the data are collected and the analyses done, then the real work starts and you face the question you have been dreading: how to write it up? This chapter looks at what is done in formal research reports, and also at three other modes of presentation – more popular articles, oral presentations and posters. The main issues are the same throughout.

A report or article or lecture has, obviously, to present the facts – what you set out to find, what you found and how you went about finding it. It has to demonstrate the **validity** of your research and its conclusions – that your research design was appropriate for the purpose and capable of sustaining the results you are claiming, that your measures or data-collection procedures validly cover what you interpret them as covering, that your interpretation of the findings is the best one available. (More to the point, the report makes it possible for other readers to test and question your research and to uncover ways in which it may not be valid and ways in which your interpretations may not be the only or the best conclusions to be drawn.) Most of all, the report has also to make interesting reading. It has to show why the research was worth doing, to tell the story of the fieldwork in an interesting manner and to grip the reader in your final discussion.

The first thing you need is an interesting title – not 'Further research on the on-ward personal interactions of a sample of male patients aged 35–45 in the county of Shropshire', but 'Interaction on the ward: a study of male patients'. However, it should be one that contains enough information to attract relevant readers (in this case 'Interaction' and 'ward/patient' are the key terms). Next in a formal report comes an Abstract, a short (200-word?) summary of what the problem is, what research was done and what the conclusions are. The final version of this is generally written last, although read first, because you can never know quite how the paper will come out until you have written it. In all research writing it is a good stratagem, however, to write a first draft of it as the first thing you write, and to keep it by you as a 'route map' to what you intend to show, a 'plot' for the story you are going to tell. Next, it is good and pleasant practice to have a brief Acknowledgements section (or to incorporate a paragraph of them into your Introduction), thanking those who have helped or advised you. Then you write yourself section headings, and within them you note very briefly what you will want to say in each section and in what order – a more detailed route map. You get your material – books you want to quote, tables or extracts from interviews, diagrams, etc. – organized for each section. Then you are ready to start.

The rest of this chapter looks at stylistic questions involved in different kinds of report writing. We cannot teach you how to write – this comes with practice. However, in our experience the business of writing is hard (but rewarding) work, so you should not be surprised if you become bored, tired or disoriented. All you can do about this is to keep writing, getting words on paper and hoping that they will 'come out right'. Getting started at all is always difficult, so the best thing once you have planned your route is to plunge straight in and start writing, even if you do not much like what you are writing. The whole paper will undoubtedly need revision before it is presentable. Most good papers go through several drafts – and the introductory paragraphs are the most likely of all the sections to need redrawing, so there is little point in trying so hard to get them right first time that you slow yourself down and do not write the rest of the paper. Get the words on paper, even if they are not the right words; revising a rough draft is easier work than writing it in the first place. (There is much to be said for using a word-processor, if you are able: redrafting becomes much easier.) Get someone else to look at and comment on your drafts, and tell them not to be afraid to be rude where necessary; you know what you wanted to get over, but it takes other people to tell you whether you succeeded and where you went wrong.

Formal reports: quantitative research

There is a traditional format which quantitative ('scientific') research reports are supposed to follow – the format which you may have used for writing up physics or chemistry experiments at school. Broadly, the report will fall into clear and labelled sections: Introduction, Methods, Results, and Discussion. The Introduction will set up the area of research and the 'problem' which is to be examined; it may, in fact, run to more than one section, if you have a lot to say and several disparate literatures to review, e.g. Introduction, The Hospital System, Research on Interaction. The Methods section says succinctly, but in enough detail that your methods can be judged by the reader, what you did. It may, again, fall into several sections if what is to be described is complex: e.g. Methods, Sampling, The Questionnaire; or Methods, The Pilot Study, Main Fieldwork. The Results section states what you found, comparatively uncritically – the results put forward as facts, and neither qualified nor commented on beyond what is necessary for an immediate understanding of them. Finally, the Discussion section will:

1 restate the findings and explain what they mean in the context of the themes you announced in your Introduction;

2 look at potential weaknesses of the methods and either discount them or argue the extent to which the results can be trusted despite these weaknesses;
3 outline the implications for the academic area and/or for policy;
4 possibly make recommendations;
5 possibly outline further research that needs to be done.

The length of the whole depends on the outlet through which you intend to publish it. Psychology journals typically publish articles of 3000–5000 words (12–20 pages of typescript, double spaced). Sociology journals expect something rather longer – typically 7000–10,000 words. Either may have a 'Brief Reports' section in which articles of not more than about 2000 words may be published. You need to look at your target publication and see what length of article they expect. An 'internal' report, for a funding authority or your own management, for example, might be of any length, but typically it would be rather fuller and more detailed than a journal article. On the other hand, it would almost certainly start with a one- or two-page section outlining the main conclusions and recommendations, for those who did not have the time or expertise to deal with the details.

In the Results section (and elsewhere, if appropriate) you will be presenting numerical information, often in the form of tables or graphs. It is important that every factual statement you make is backed up with figures, and unless the figures are very simple indeed – e.g. a comparison of two percentages or two means – it will be appropriate to present them in tabular form. The tables which are presented in the text should form part of the argument and should be extremely simple and readable – as simple as it as possible to be and still make the desired point. There may be a case for presenting more complex figures from which other researchers can check your conclusions or carry out further analysis, but such 'storehouse' tables should usually be in an Appendix, not in the main text. At the same time you should remember that no set of figures speaks for itself, and you should always interpret the results in words as well as giving the figures. Each stage of the argument in the Results section has the same structure:

1 what is to be shown;
2 how it is to be shown;
3 table or description of results;
4 what it means.

The other requirement, in this kind of research, is that no conclusion should go untested. Wherever you present a result – a difference, or a **correlation**, or some other relationship – you should also present an associated test of significance (unless the result is so small or so large that it clearly does not need testing). You need to show that what you are stating as 'fact' is not a chance product of sampling variation, so tests of statistical significance are absolutely required. (Again you should interpret them in words; you cannot safely assume that all your readers will understand them – particularly if your report is for management or for a funding body.) Even when comparing figures not at first sight based on samples – e.g. the actual numbers of cases processed in two different years – it may still be appropriate to test for significance, treating the two years as random samples from all the years you could possibly have examined and looking for indications of more than chance variation between them.

An important point to remember is that any explicit or implicit promises of confidentiality or anonymity that you have made should be honoured. It is important that your informants should not be identifiable from your report unless they have explicitly stated that their names may be given. To preserve confidentiality may mean going beyond suppressing names, to omitting or changing (fictionalizing) identifiable circumstances.

Formal reports: qualitative research

Qualitative research reports – reports of open interviewing projects and/or open or participant observation – do not generally follow this set structure. Researchers of this kind do not generally think of themselves as scientists, and they have no desire to emulate the report of the scientific experiment. However, just the same topics and sections have to be covered in the report. You still have:

1 to introduce your field of research and explain why it is interesting;
2 to explain what you did, and how;
3 to give the results;
4 to interpret them and qualify them.

There is more leeway to 'tell the story', but you still have to demonstrate that what you did was a valid way of researching the problem or area you elected to tackle, and that your interpretation of what was said to you and what you saw is a valid one. Thus without having the same formal sub-headings, you may well find yourself falling into the same general structure.

The presentation of data will necessarily be more impressionistic in this kind of report. Where statements are being made about *numbers* of people who do or say something, tables may still be appropriate, and certainly numbers are better than vague impressions: '60 per cent of the sample' or '90 per cent' carries more conviction and is more interpretable than 'many' or 'a majority'. Often, however, you will be making points about interviews that could be fully substantiated only by reproducing the entire transcript, which is not practical for reasons of length and because the point would still not emerge until the reader had put as much time into analysis as you have done. One therefore makes points and illustrates them with pertinent quotations from the transcript. One or two quotations do not constitute compelling evidence, but they give a feel for what the informant actually said and allow the reader to try interpreting it in some different way.

A key aspect of validating qualitative research is **reflexivity** – showing at each stage of the report that you have a reasonable grasp of what went on, how you were seen and construed by the informant(s), and the extent to which your own preconceptions, theoretical frame or professional status may have interacted with the data and your interpretation of it. Hitting the right degree of reflexivity is difficult. If your report reads too much like a diary of your feelings and experiences and is too dominated by 'I', 'me' and 'my', it will annoy or embarrass the reader. On the other hand, this kind of research is mediated through the person of the researcher, and we need to find out about that person in order to understand and trust the results. This is very much a case for showing your first draft to someone else – preferably someone experienced in this kind of research – to see if you have hit the right level.

In reports of this kind of research we need to remember that it is the detail that carries conviction, but that the detail is also what can betray the identity of the informants. Particular care must be exercised that people are not 'exposed' in this way, so fictional names are normally given to informants and it is often necessary to suppress or even fictionalize some of the details, or to 'add two cases together', in order not to publish the intimate details of an identifiable individual's life.

Other modes of presentation

Quite often what you are called on to write is not a formal research report, but a 'popular account', by which we mean anything from an account for the general public to an article in a professional journal aimed more at practice than research (e.g. *Nursing Times*, *Social Work Today*). The same considerations come into play – you must still give enough detail of how the research was carried out that its validity can be judged by the informed reader. However, the 'slant' will necessarily be different, more towards why the area is interesting and how your results contribute to it, and less towards the detail of the research procedures. You can allow yourself a greater degree of speculation and 'following up ideas' in a popular account than would be normal in a formal report. However, you should never state as fact (or imply to be true) what you have not established, and you should be very careful about overgeneralizing your results and claiming for the research an importance which it does not bear.

A more difficult task which you may well be called on to perform if you have carried out research is to make an oral presentation – a lecture, or a short presentation, to a public audience or your peers or to management or those who have commissioned or funded the research. The same principles apply, but your presentation has to be less dense, with only the important highlights brought out. You would be surprised how little can be delivered in a given amount of time when you present your results orally. You will be lucky to get one 'point' across in five minutes in a compressed and 'slick' session such as a market-research presentation, and in the more relaxed and didactic setting of a lecture one point in ten minutes would be more realistic. This means that you can only say five or six things in an hour's lecture, and you have to be very careful and self-disciplined in selecting the six points that you want to make.

Time is saved, and the pace of the presentation is more enjoyable for the audience, if you use pre-prepared visual aids such as slides for an overhead projector. These can be used to present tables and diagrams, and also to summarize lists to points in a memorable form. Photocopied hand-outs can also be used, to deliver material which it is essential for the audience to receive, but which does not fit easily within the ambit of the lecture (i.e. detailed tables or details of controversial aspects of the research process).

Finally, at conferences and other situations where research results are exchanged, there is a growing fashion for 'poster' presentation – researchers delivering their results in visual form, often literally on one poster (but being present to discuss them with anyone whom the poster attracts). The skill here, obviously, is the skill of abstract-writing – working out the absolute minimum that needs to be displayed, and presenting it in a graphic and arresting form (with at least some important part of it read-able from a distance). You can make even fewer points than in a lecture, and they have to be made in a very few words or, preferably, pictorially. Sometimes cartoons can be used to advantage. For an example of a research project whose report was presented in this way, see the article 'Doing dia-logical research' by Rosemary Randall and John Southgate, in Reason and Rowan (1981).

Exercise 37: Writing up

If you would like to, why not take one of the small pieces of research you carried out in connection with Chapter 1 – perhaps the structured and unstructured observation – and try writing it up? (Look at some examples of reports first – see below.) Aim for something quite short – 2000 words at most. Get someone familiar with research to look over it and comment on it for you. Then think how you could boil it down to (a) a 20-minute oral presentation, and (b) a poster display.

Summary

1 A formal report has to present the results, show how they were collected and what may validly be concluded from them and, more important, what may *not* validly be concluded. At the same time it has to interest the reader and show why the research was worth doing and the conclusions are worth considering.

2 Quantitative/scientific reports tend to follow a set format – Introduction (what is being investigated, and why), Methods (how the research was done), Results (what was found) and Discussion (what it means). The whole is not an autobiography of research experience but a logical argu-ment running from questions at the start to conclusions at the end, via interpreted research results and arguments supporting the interpretation.

3 Qualitative research reports are more varied in form, but they still have the same kind of argument to present and so the same material will have to be covered.

Further reading

For examples of quantitative reports, see the three articles by Gordon, Abbott and Tyler, and Doll and Hill, in Abbott and Sapsford (eds) (1997) *Research into Practice: A Reader for Nurses and the Caring Professions* (2nd edition). The Gordon article is probably the best to use as a model, in terms of structure.

For examples of qualitative reports, see the articles by Kirkham, Cayne, and Abbott and Sapsford, in the same book.

CHAPTER FIFTEEN

IN CONCLUSION: RESEARCH INTO PRACTICE

In this final chapter we try to bring together the main threads of the argument, to look at the contribution research has to make to professional practice and its relationship to the evaluation of practice and policy. Much of
the book has been about evaluation in one form or another, and all of the
methods and styles we have discussed could have a part to play. It is
important, however, to make a distinction between *methods* – the design
and techniques we use when we are carrying out research – and the *pur-
poses/reasons* for doing the research. Insofar as it has an existence separate
from other kinds of research, evaluation research is **applied** – research
undertaken to solve a problem or, more accurately, to see if the hypothe-
sized solution to a problem is working. However, it can also be **strategic**:
that is, the findings can (and, if published, will) be generalized beyond the
particular case. The findings are also likely to contribute to **theory** – to the
ways in which we make sense of and explain what is going on. All research
into practice or policy has some element of the applied or at least the
strategic, but good research is also concerned with a wider understanding
beyond the particular case and a wider context within which to make sense
of the results.

We also need, in this final chapter, to look beyond techniques of research
again, to what lies *behind* the research which you carry out or read about.
Research is seldom or never carried out just 'to collect the facts' in some
supposedly neutral way. Behind the research project lies the hypothesis to
be tested, the theory to be extended or clarified, the problem to be solved,
the policy to be evaluated, the practice to be improved or monitored. Even
the **Census** is not a totally neutral piece of data collection; the questions
which are chosen are there because answers are needed, for planning
schools, hospitals, local services, etc. We may divide research projects and
programmes, crudely, into those which are aimed at the development and
elucidation of theory ('academic research') and those which are aimed at

solving a practical problem, or developing or monitoring a social policy, or assessing and improving how professionals or others do their jobs ('applied research'). This chapter is structured as if the divide between these two kinds of research were an absolute one. As we shall see, however, theory and practice interpenetrate – theory has consequences, and practice is based explicitly or implicitly on theory.

Research-based practice

The book has been half about how to carry out research, but half about how to read the reports of other people's research and take from them what has been validly established. The evaluation of practice through research is central to what it is agreed is needed for the development of the 'caring trades' – nursing, for example – into true professions and their practitioners into autonomous professionals: the development of research-based practice. However, Boon (1995) has indicated that research-developed practice is *not* currently being achieved in nursing. She argues that nurses continue to support practices and developments which have no sound research base; sometimes they continue with some that research has shown to be detrimental to patients. Hunt (1981) suggested a number of reasons why research is not put into practice; these included a lack of knowledge of research findings, a lack of understanding of them, a lack of trust in them, a lack of knowledge as to how to implement the findings in practice, and opposition by nurse managers to the findings being implemented. She goes on to suggest that researchers share some of the blame for research findings not being used. Problems include the production of findings that do not make utilization possible, researchers not studying the problems of practitioners, and researchers not explaining the value of their findings convincingly.

If nursing is to develop as a research-based profession, two things will be necessary. Both nurses and the organizations in which they are employed will need to be determined that practice shall be based on research/knowledge. At the same time, relevant research will have to be carried out, directed at the problems/issues of practice and written up in an accessible and usable form. This does not mean that all nurses have to carry out research (although all nurses should reflect on practice), but it does require that nurses have the skills to evaluate and implement the findings of research carried out by others. It also requires that nurses shall be able to justify their practices by reference to relevant, well designed and well executed research – that practice is informed by research findings. Nursing procedures and practice should be informed by research just as medical treatment is. We expect, for example, that research, including **controlled trials**, will be carried out before new drugs are introduced. We also expect that the research that is carried out will be of high quality. This is equally crucial for nursing research (and research within any other of the caring professions).

However, it is necessary to avoid blind faith in research. Research is necessary but not sufficient as a basis for practice, and it is necessary to be reflective and to evaluate the research findings in the context of practice. In the past, for example, new drugs have been introduced after controlled trials, but the long-term effects have not been evaluated; the contraceptive pill is one example here. Further, nursing is a social act, and the social and political consequences of treatment are often as relevant as the clinical consequences; nurses need to work *with* patients rather than *on* them. Quality of life may be preferred to quantity of life by some patients. Decisions may have to be made about appropriate treatment when there are conflicting interests. Ann Oakley's research on pregnancy and childbirth, for example, indicated that doctors saw a healthy mother and baby as the defining characteristics of a successful outcome. Mothers, on the other hand, were also concerned with the social and emotional aspects; they were dissatisfied with medical care because they felt that they were treated as objects to be worked on.

Ethical issues are another important aspect of the evaluation of research: the question of the extent to which it is ethically and politically acceptable to implement research findings. For example, in the early twentieth century research seemed to support the view that mild mental subnormality was hereditable. Suggested ways to prevent it being passed on included life-long segregation and sterilization. In the United States and a number of European countries legislation was passed for the mandatory sterilization of people with mild learning difficulties, but it was regarded as unacceptable in Britain (Abbott and Sapsford 1987b).

Another aspect is the issue of preferred outcomes. Research may suggest that a given treatment may have both positive and negative outcomes. An example would be hormone replacement therapy for menopausal women, which has potential beneficial effects and potentially harmful side effects. Informed consent may be an important issue: giving patients the necessary information so that they can be involved in decisions about their treatment. Wendy Savage – a consultant gynaecologist – argued for women to be informed about potential outcomes so that they could make choices about how they gave birth; she encountered considerable resistance from her male colleagues (Savage 1986). An additional issue here was the question of whose interests should be prioritized: those of the mother or those of the unborn child. However, it is not only with respect to unborn children that research may indicate different treatment depending on whose interests are prioritized. Psychological research suggests that children, especially young children, need the care of their mothers, while other research suggests that women are less likely to suffer mental health problems if they have paid employment (Abbott and Wallace 1996).

Basing practice on research, then, requires careful evaluation of the research to assess its **validity** and **reliability**. It also requires a consideration of ethical and political issues and a recognition that patients are people to be worked with and not objects to be worked on. In addition it requires that practitioners reflect on – critically review – their own practice. What nurses and other caring professionals can bring to their reading of research – and their conduct of it – is an 'insider perspective' which is different from that of the other professionals with whom they associate and reflects the internal logic of their practice. In the health field, for example, the nursing perspective can be clearly differentiated from the medical one.

Doctors do research on leg ulcers, for example, but nurses are naturally concerned with the patient who has leg ulcers and how he or she is to deal with the condition along with the other demands of everyday life. Medical research is concerned with successful pregnancy, but nurses, midwives and health visitors listen to pregnant women and can come to understand the part of children and childbirth in their lives as a whole, and they may therefore come to a rather different definition of 'success' in some cases. The professional stance in the caring professions, and thus in the research associated with them, involves understanding lives and reducing problems, rather than isolating and treating 'conditions'.

Not all of the research relevant to the professions will be carried out *by* professionals. In health, for example, much medical research is relevant to nurse and health visitor practice, as is wider sociological 'social policy' and psychological research into structural inequalities in health and poverty, authority relations, doctor–patient interactions and 'social problems' (e.g. 'battered child syndrome', or 'domestic violence'). Some research into practice will be carried out by academic researchers, or employed researchers, who bring an 'outsider perspective' and a different body of disciplinary knowledge to bear on practitioner problems; the 'professional stranger' may have much to contribute simply by being able to take an unanticipated perspective on familiar problems and practices. Much research into practice will be carried out by practitioners, however, who know from the inside what the problems and possibilities are likely to be and how to present the results most usefully to their fellow professionals. Indeed, much research into practice – seldom written up as formal reports – involves practitioners and groups of practitioners trying to rationalize and improve *their own* practice. Thus many different kinds of research, carried out by many different kinds of researcher, can form the basis of research-based practice.

Evaluating practice

When we talk about evaluation we tend to think of set-piece 'studies', probably quantitative and 'scientific' in nature, which explore the effects of some policy change or innovation in practice. Other kinds of evaluation study are possible and sometimes more appropriate, however. Despite policy-makers' known predilection for the quantitative and scientific, studies using more open or qualitative methods have been gaining ground in the last 20 years, for example. There is also a great deal that can be done in the way of evaluating one's own practice without ever starting anything as formal as 'an evaluation study'.

In industrial processes, one research-like activity which happens as a matter of routine is *quality control* – testing the product, before sale, to ensure that it is fit for its purpose. Sometimes, where the testing is cheap and easy, it can be done on every single item: hotels make a quick visual check of all bedrooms, after they have been cleaned, before reletting them. Sometimes every item has to be checked even if the testing is expensive and adds to the price of the goods. Computers are individually tested before sale, for example, and if the computer is to run a telephone exchange or to form part of a surgical procedure then the testing can be extensive and take days. Most often, however, testing is done on a sample of the product. When testing light bulbs, for example, a small sample of each batch is tested to destruction. If the results are satisfactory, the batch is passed. If they are not, then a larger sample will be examined to see if the first result was due to chance – several failures in a sample may have come from a batch of goods which in fact contains no higher a proportion of defective bulbs than is considered acceptable. Statistical theory can be used to determine what size of sample should be taken in order to work to given probability of revealing that a batch is flawed.

In the same way, we all monitor our practice informally – we note where we have performed unsatisfactorily and resolve to do better – but the reflective practitioner can use the 'research imagination' to do this more formally and rigorously. In some circumstances, where any kind of failure is totally unacceptable, detailed records are kept of every case and are studied after the event to yield pointers for future performance. Some surgical procedures are recorded on video, for example, and the video carefully examined. Follow-up examination would also be undertaken, to monitor outcome not just at the 'point of delivery' but months or even years after apparent success. Even in less crucial cases record-keeping is a key to improved performance. The records of particular cases can be scanned, for example to ensure that no sloppiness or bad practice is creeping into the treatment routine. Records of 'successful' cases can be compared *en bloc* with records of 'unsuccessful' ones, to detect similarities or differences. Indeed, records of particular *kinds* of cases can be examined as a whole, once sufficient have been accumulated, to look for similarities and differences of condition, note what the practitioner actually did and compare outcomes. This is the usual form of 'research' carried out by many psychologists and therapists, looking back over past case records to spot patterns and make recommendations for their own and others' future practice.

If you are carrying out a formal 'evaluation study' of a policy or procedure, in the scientific style, the important thing is rigour of design and execution, so that you can argue plausibly from the results as to the success (or otherwise) of what you were testing. You will need, first, to specify the treatment as clearly as possible in procedural terms, and to specify the outcome – what will count as 'success' and what as unacceptable failure. What you are looking for as outcome will of course depend on the cost of the procedure and the importance of the area of study. In the case of a cheap procedure which might have an effect on death rates, for example, you would be inclined to count as success *any* indication that the procedure might be effective. Where the procedure was expensive to administer you would need a clearer indication that the expense was worthwhile, particularly if the condition to be treated was something relatively minor, a nuisance rather than a threat. (We have cast this discussion in medical terms, but just the same holds for evaluations of housing policy or income maintenance.) Having determined the 'treatment' and what is to count as outcome, you need to **operationalize** your variables – to translate them into something directly countable or measurable – and probably to build in checks on the reliability and validity of the measures. If possible you will want a comparison group to run alongside the treatment group, to strengthen the causal element in your argument – and you will need to demonstrate that the groups are comparable. (If random allocation to treatment and **control groups** is not possible it may be necessary to compare with another naturally occurring group or with what happened in the past; in this case it will be all the more important to demonstrate that there are not large differences between the group undergoing treatment and those with whom you intend to compare them.) You will need to show that the groups with which you are working are likely to be **representative** of the populations to which you want to generalize the results, and an element of **random** sampling and/or random allocation will normally be appropriate here. You will want to collect information on anything else which might be of importance to your eventual argument. You will want to start your measurements before instituting the treatment or change, and if possible continue them after the treatment has ended, to put a **longitudinal** component into the argument. In other words, you will need to anticipate all possible objections to your results and guard against them in the design and conduct of the research. (In practice you will not be able to do so – 'real-world' research is often flawed, because of the intransigence of real situations. Further, there may often be grave ethical objections to what research design would suggest are correct procedures; random allocation to treatments, for example, is often not ethically acceptable. However, you will need to be as rigorous as you can in the circumstances which you face.)

This kind of research, if properly constructed, is very strong as a way of testing causal hypotheses – well grounded theories about what ought to work or how things ought to be done. Where it is *not* strong, however, is in the breadth of opportunity it gives the researcher to formulate *fresh* theory and take a different slant on things – the respondent's/informant's slant. A well designed quantitative evaluation study can offer reasonably firm conclusions, but it is caught in the theoretical stance which informs its design – it can deliver new knowledge, but seldom or never new theory. For research which is open not just to confirming or denying the efficacy of a treatment or policy but to entirely rethinking how we view the condition which is being treated or dealt with, qualitative approaches are required. This is nowhere more evident than in feminist research on pregnancy and childbirth. There is a great deal of scientific research on the reproduction process, leading to more efficacious treatments, to the control of pain and to the more certain survival of infants born in difficult circumstances, and we would not wish in any way to decry such work. It took a generation of feminist scholars, however, working initially from and with women's vague discontent with 'the way things were' when they had their babies, to question the dominant medical paradigm and point out that it is *not* necessary to consider pregnancy as a disease on a par with tuberculosis or hernia – something which doctors and medicine are to monitor and 'cure'. Women's own experience, as revealed in open interview studies and confirmed in **participant observation**, was that they were treated as medical machines, or as sick persons, and subject to the near-absolute control of medical men and medical technology. To argue that something better is possible for women – that they can make more sense of this fraught stage of their lives than just as a medical problem to be solved by someone else – it was necessary to use qualitative means of data collection, for only so could such evidence be obtained in a form where it might convince those who are in a position to change policy and practice.

Qualitative, 'open' methods are more and more used in research into social policy and professional practice, and are becoming increasingly acceptable to administrators and policy-makers. This is at least in part due to the growing realization among those who read such reports that 'open' research is not something formless, subjective and 'wishy-washy', but subject to the same degree of rigour as more quantitative studies (as we have seen in earlier chapters). Just as much care and thought has to be put into demonstrating that the informants or actors are **typical** of the population to be considered, that the procedures are well designed to elicit genuine information rather than just responses specific to the context of research, and that the researcher's biases and preconceptions do not dominate the analysis of the data. Indeed, in three respects such research may be seen as *more* rigorous than quantitative studies:

1 much more thought tends to be put into the interview or observation context as a social situation into which the researcher as well as the researched makes an input and which has a *meaning* for the informant/actor which crucially affects the data which are collected;
2 because the possibilities of falsifying or overenthusiastically interpreting data are patently so much greater in qualitative work, a tradition has grown up within it of much more open and politically/ethically/**ideologically** explicit writing on the part of the researcher, trying not to conceal but to identify possible sources of bias and preconception; and
3 even **critical/discourse research** tends to experience a duty to put across the informants' point of view, in the informants' own words and concepts, whatever else these words may be used to demonstrate, so a 'duty of openness' is imposed on the research in a way which, as we have said, is not always the case with quantitative studies.

Increasingly it has been argued that **action research** is the core method of nursing research, in the same way the clinical controlled trial is for medical research. However, there is confusion in the literature as to what action research *is*. The essence of 'action research', it seems to us – what makes it a distinctive approach – is that it arises out of practice and feeds back into practice. We would use the term for evaluative studies which are not extraneous to what is being evaluated but built into the design of the policy or practice, or at least successfully woven into it *post hoc*. Distinctively, action research in the nursing professions is aimed at the continual improvement of practice and therefore at being directly applicable, and it is typically (though not *necessarily*) carried out by the practitioners themselves. In its general use, the term 'action research' does not necessarily imply qualitative work; any kind of research style may form a part of it. When directed at the problems of caring practice, however, it very often does involve a qualitative framework, because (as we argued above) caring practitioners tend towards the kind of **holistic** and **naturalistic** approach to the framing of problems which tends to demand open interviewing and observation rather than the **reductionist** logic of **experimental** or **survey** methods.

Practitioner research has been described as central to the development of nursing theory and practice and to nurses as autonomous practitioners; the same may be said for any other of the caring professions. Practice based on research can be seen as *accountable* practice. Increasingly it has been argued that the reflective approach is central to research in nursing and other caring professions. The movement towards greater collaboration in research is one example of a wider process which we might call a move towards 'the reflective researcher'. The reflective practitioner is one who uses the research imagination on his or her professional practice, analysing performance and the reactions to performance – and the ethical presuppositions and models of the person and society in which it is grounded – and attempts to improve. Under the influence of qualitative researchers and the scholarly critiques provided by feminists, anti-racist writers and the disability rights movement, researchers are coming to apply this same question to their own practice and to question some of the taken-for-granted assumptions and power relations which it involves.

The force of the 'collaborative' notion, and its appeal for action researchers, lies partly in a critique of both of the two models according to which conventional research is conducted. In *academic research*, however noble the aims of the researcher, the research can very fairly be described as being in the interests of the researcher: he or she does it to retain an academic job, to obtain promotion, to 'improve the curriculum vitae' when it comes to looking for jobs, or for the glory (and, very occasionally, the financial profit) of being published. *Employed research* is generally done in the interests of a customer: the research team is employed to find a solution to a problem. Both kinds of research are fairly charged with using people as objects: the subjects of the research are raw material for academic analysis or commercial or management exploitation. Increasingly, under the influence of both humanistic psychologists and feminists, researchers are turning to a more collaborative way of working.

The classic '**collaborative research**' of those who advocate it as an alternative way of working which shares power more evenly, requires researchers and other participants to combine together to solve some problem which is of importance to the participants; research reports emerge as a by-product rather than the main aim. The most collaborative of all research designs comes from the area of psychotherapy, with the concept of co-counselling. Concerned with the power inequality implicit in the therapeutic relationship, some counsellors have adopted a procedure whereby both parties to a therapeutic interview are regarded equally as counsellor and as client – that is, the problems of both are explored, and each attempts to deliver help to the other (see Jackins 1965). On some occasions, jointly written research reports have emerged from such projects. Similar approaches have been taken to the assessment and appraisal of professional performance. Teachers, for example, have entered into 'mutual evaluation contracts' whereby they appraised each other's classroom performance and enabled each other to see what they looked like when seen through other eyes; similar collaborative evaluations have been carried out in the medical profession and in management (see Heron 1977, 1979, 1981). As a feedback method it has great advantages, the chief being that the assessment is not carried out by some outsider standing in a position of potential power over the subject of the appraisal, but by involved colleagues who are themselves to be appraised by the same process.

A second collaborative model is that of the researcher, as researcher or as social scientist, joining a group's efforts to obtain some shared goal – and, in the process, writing up the struggle towards that goal as a report of research – collaborative action research. Many of the good examples are feminist. For example, Maria Mies and a group of other sociologists, all active in the women's movement, helped to obtain a shelter for battered women in Cologne and went on, with the collaboration of those who came to the shelter, to explore women's experiences of being wives under these circumstances (Mies 1983). This differs from the examples above in that the researchers were not directly dealing with a problem which they shared – they had not themselves been in such a relationship (one presumes) – but they made the problem their own and worked along with those who did have direct experience of it to deal with the practical difficulties and the emotional problems experienced by the latter.

Not infrequently you will find a piece of research described as co-research whose declared aim is 'facilitation' – helping people to see their situation for what it is. Many feminist papers are of this kind, and some interactional work inspired by a Marxist viewpoint which seeks to teach people about their working situation and the direction in which their interests 'really' lie. Some more humanistic work can also be described in these terms. Note, however, that this kind of 'facilitation' is not collaborative in the same way as co-research or collaborative appraisal. It does not exhibit the same equality of power and ownership; on the contrary, its essence is that of one group (researchers) changing or working on another group (subjects/participants). Similar **rhetoric** does not necessarily guarantee similarly structured research. The research by Julia Cayne into nurse education and professional development which we looked at earlier is another example of collaborative work where the goals may be said to be set by the group leader and only imperfectly shared by the 'collaborators'; development is clearly a goal of the nurses, and they collaborate with the tutor to reach this goal, but learning to develop by this particular method is something perhaps *imposed* on them.

To sum up: practice may be evaluated by any of the many methods of research discussed in this book, but *caring* practice lends itself particularly to qualitative and collaborative evaluation – colleagues getting together to examine their practice, or researchers 'in the field' getting together with clients to help solve the problems of daily living and examine how they may best be solved in everyone's interests. Even where there is no true collaboration, there will generally be an openness to the views of those who form the subjects of research, and generally the research and its aims will be discussed with them. The professional stance of the caring professions is generally a holistic one, and so good evaluative research into caring practice will generally take the perspective of the 'subject' and be to some extent 'insider' research rather than just external, 'objective' observation. Studies of the problems of clients may be 'one-off' projects, but evaluation of professional practice may more often require 'action research' – a continuing circle of research feeding back into practice, which in turn modifies the research.

The reflective researcher

As we argued in the first chapter of this book, the essence of research is not technique – though techniques are important – but imagination. Increasingly it has been argued that the reflective approach is central to research in nursing. The movement towards greater openness and collaboration in research is one example of a wider process which we might call a move towards 'the reflective researcher'. The reflective practitioner is one who uses the research imagination on his or her professional practice, analysing performance and the reactions to performance – and the ethical presuppositions and models of the person and society in which it is grounded – and attempts to improve.

Insightful imagination – the reflexive stance – is needed in every kind of research, from the immediate evaluation of one's own practice up to large-scale fact-finding exercises on which policy will be based. It is always necessary to specify the 'problem' with great care, to define with precision the goal of the policy or practice or innovation, and to specify what shall count as a favourable or unfavourable outcome. In thinking about outcomes it is necessary to use a great deal of imagination, to get beyond the formal 'declaration of purpose' and think how the policy-makers or practitioners will react to various kinds of outcome which they have not yet envisaged. The same applies when you are setting out to evaluate your own practice. It is necessary also to think carefully about the way that the research is framed and the way in which you intend to carry it out, to see who might be hurt or unsettled by it and whose interests might be harmed.

Assessing a new way of nursing certain patients, for instance, the declared goal will undoubtedly be to improve the health or speed the recovery of the patients; we are all in favour of honour and virtue, and the virtuous nurse works towards the good of the patients. Thinking of what outcomes would be *acceptable*, however, we would probably feel that the technique was worth introducing if it made the patients more comfortable, or even if they just preferred it to the previous way of working, even if it had no measurable effect on health. We might even think it worth introducing if all it did was to make the nurse's job easier or more pleasant, provided the patients were no worse off than before. So an acceptable outcome may be something substantially less than would be implied by the rhetoric of treatment. We have also to consider the constraints on acceptability. If we carried out research on a nursing treatment and found it had a measurable effect on speed of recovery, we might declare the treatment a success. Would it be adopted, however, if it cost a great deal more than the previous treatment? Or if it meant substantially increasing the establishment of nursing staff? Or if it meant a great deal more work for the nurses who implemented it? *How much* extra cost, in money or staff or time, would be acceptable? In other words, is the goal better formulated as 'to speed recovery, or to make patients more comfortable, *at little or no extra cost*'? Indeed, might it be true (as often appears the case at the time of writing) that the real goal is to reduce costs, with the constraint being that patients must not be much worse off and nurses not much more hard-pressed in their jobs? The true goals of policy-makers (or your own, looking at your own practice) may not be as honourable and virtuous as the usual rhetoric may suggest.

The difference between rhetoric and reality is well worth bearing in mind when reading other people's research. Sometimes you will find that apparent lapses of logic – rejecting conclusions on less than adequate grounds, or jumping to conclusions as 'obvious' which seem less than obvious to you – may betray a 'hidden agenda' influenced by what is implicitly counted as an adequate outcome or implicitly acknowledged as a constraint on the acceptability of an outcome, without the writer having explicitly stated what is affecting his or her judgement. Indeed, you may occasionally come across a report which quite blatantly reinterprets the evidence, intending not to assess whether current practice fits the declared aims, but to show how the declared aims can be reinterpreted to fit current practice. The status quo often attracts very powerful defensive manoeuvres.

An important part of 'research imagination' is seeing beyond what one tends to take for granted, looking for different ways of doing what has always been done in a particular way, even questioning whether the reasons why it is done are still beyond questioning. One is reminded of one of the early 'time and motion' studies, carried out on gun-teams in the French army before the Second World War. The researchers worked out what each person in the team was supposed to be doing while the gun was being readied, and it turned out that the entire job of one team member was to hold the officer's horse. French artillery officers had not been mounted for several years by this time.

The ethical status of research is an important area of operation for the reflective imagination. We have talked about ethics throughout this book mainly in terms of avoiding harm to 'subjects', and the question of the extent to which it is legitimate to deceive people and/or use them as 'objects'. The question of deception is a difficult one in any kind of research on and for people which is not fully collaborative. In principle we would say that it is not legitimate to carry out research without the full and informed consent of those who are affected, and this principle is written into the ethical codes of many of the professional associations. In practice, however, the codified principle does not solve all of the ethical problems.

1 Sometimes – as in some controlled trials – the research would become ineffective if the 'subjects' were alerted beforehand to what was going on, because of **reactivity**.

2 Sometimes there cannot be full and informed consent because the informants will not understand the implications of the research, not having the same background, training and goals as the researchers; for example, to what extent can informants really give *informed* consent to a **psychometric questionnaire** study investigating the psychological bases of clinical depression and its antecedents in everyday life.

3 Sometimes asking for consent might itself be harmful or unsettling – in the depression study, for example, explaining the goals might amount to saying 'We're going to give you this questionnaire which will measure whether you're likely to go mad.'

4 *Whose* consent is needed is not always obvious. In the case of research on

institutionalized older people, for example, do we need the consent of
the older people themselves, or the staff of the residential homes, or their
managers, or the medical personnel, or the older people's relatives, or
...? Research Ethics Committees are likely to require that you obtain the
informed written consent of relatives/legal guardians where subjects
cannot provide it themselves – children, confused elderly people, people
with severe learning difficulties. Your wider ethics, however, may require
you also to inform participants themselves and to try to do so in a way
which enables them to make sense of what is going on.

5 Finally, there are some cases where research on the powerful or the con-
spiratorial may mean deliberate deception. You will not get much by way
of results, in research into 'insider trading' on the stock market, by asking
people whether they have ever committed this particular criminal
offence. Open and consensual research into brutality in institutions or
by the police is not likely to produce much in the way of useful results.
These dramatic examples make the problem look simple, but it remains
an ethical dilemma because the justification for deception and 'spying'
lies with the judgement of the researcher. And there can be more subtle
problems, on a smaller scale. For example, suppose (something we are
sure is highly unlikely, but *suppose*) that a nurse's research were turned
down by a Research Ethics Committee and he or she was sure the major
reason was to prevent nuisance or embarrassment to doctors or hospital
administrators; would there then be justification for 'going under-
ground' and carrying out the research in secret?

Ethical questions also stretch to the perspective from which the research
is undertaken. As a practitioner, or as a researcher commissioned by 'management', one naturally feels that the purposes of the system under investigation and the way in which it is run are in the interests of
patients/clients/recipients. It is possible, however, that the way these interests are perceived are management-defined, and that the people themselves might define their interests in quite different ways. A case in point is
the way in which contraceptive advice is given to Black women. We generally accept as liberal and beneficial that advice on contraceptives be made
freely available to working-class women. Sometimes Black women feel,
however, that the advice is aimed mainly at controlling their fertility
because of White middle-class fears, and sometimes the evidence suggests
that they are right (see Bryan *et al.* 1985 for a discussion).

The question of neutrality in research is not an easy one. Clearly, the
researcher should not take sides to the extent that the research becomes
polemic and results contrary to the researcher's position cannot emerge.
We might also argue, however, that one role of social research is to make
space for the voices to be heard of those who do not usually get a hearing.
Since the 1970s academic researchers have been asking 'Whose side are we
on?' and have advocated research not into the control of crime or the
explanation of poverty or unemployment but the experience of impover-
ished and disadvantaged people and their needs and legitimate desires.
Similarly, those who speak for disadvantaged groups have advocated
research not into the groups as problems but into the problems of the
groups: feminists do research on women's subordination and the ways of

alleviating it, and the disabled rights movement looks not at how disabled people can be fitted into the everyday world but at how the everyday world can be changed to accommodate them and give them full rights as citizens. If researchers do not in some sense 'speak for the underdog' then it is not clear who will do so (nor why 'the underdog' should tolerate being researched). A part of research reflectivity also involves being aware of the political, ethical and ideological stances which underlie the theories which give rise to research, and the political uses of apparently neutral methods and results. At a more mundane level, it involves an awareness that research *is* a political activity and that the results will be used in some group's interests to dominate, disadvantage, control or at least predict the behaviour of some other group.

The nature of research as an activity has also been profoundly questioned in recent years. As we pointed out above, research is in the first instance an activity undertaken in the interests of the researcher – to 'make' professional esteem, money, promotion, etc. – and this shows very clearly in the mode of operation of the typical researcher, whose work is

> conducted on a rape model: the researchers take, hit and run. They intrude into their subjects' privacy, disrupt their perceptions, utilise false pretences, manipulate the relationship, and give little or nothing in return. When the needs of the researchers are satisfied, they break off contact with the subject.
>
> (Reinharz 1979: 95)

Even where full collaboration is not feasible, or where the researcher does not wish to adopt a collaborative stance, there is an increasing awareness that researchers have no *right* to their data – that they are beggars and intruders. Increasingly, we are asked (and asking)

1 whether the research is necessary and justified – whether, for example, the likely results of a survey of women sexually abused by their fathers is worth the pain and distress which it might cause;
2 whether the particular researcher has any right to be carrying out the particular research – whether, for example, it is a part of the researcher's work as a counsellor of such women, or just something chosen because it is a 'sexy' topic and would make a good article or dissertation, and
3 what is in it for the informants – whether they (or their group in general) benefit in any way from the research, or whether all the benefits that accrue are to the researchers and/or their customers/sponsors.

Research and theory

By 'theory' in this section we shall mean not the particular theory (derived perhaps from sociology or social psychology) which a programme of research might be designed to test, but underlying perspectives or models (of the social order and the nature of people and institutions within it) which are expressed in the way the research is conceptualized. Again, we are looking critically at what is taken for granted, assumed or posited as a natural or sensible way of conceptualizing the world within which the research problem is set.

Models of the social world differ widely. You may conceptualize the social order in a 'functionalist' way, influenced knowingly or unknowingly by theorists such as Merton and Parsons, and conceive of society as a relatively coherent whole sharing a large measure of agreement as to what is normal and how things should be, but with small pockets of deviants at the outskirts who do not or cannot share that consensus. In that case your conception of the research problem is likely to be influenced by the notion that every social structure has a function – by definition, because in this view a structure which was not functional would not survive – and be interested in working out what that function was. (The concept of 'the sick role' is a typical functionalist notion.) You may hold an essentially Marxist or 'conflict theory' model of society, seeing the social order as riven with economic inequalities, and social structures as set up to maintain and promote the position of the dominant class (those who own or control the means of production). Concepts of ideology are natural in this perspective, and the sort of research that follows from it demonstrates differential health chances by class, or differential use of and benefit from health resources; some of the best research on third world countries and the role of multinational drug companies in exploiting markets within them has also been influenced by this perspective. You may find yourself with an essentially individualistic model of the social order, which denies the existence of 'society' or 'social structures' and attempts to explain everything in terms of the interactions of individuals. In addition, or instead, you may be influenced by one of a variety of feminist perspectives, all of which stress the concept of patriarchy or patriarchal relations – the structural and/or personal domination of women by men. Each of these ways of looking at social relations has its impact on how you conceptualize research into the health and personal social services, which lie at an important point of intersection between different theories. How they are conceptualized affects not only how they are expected to function, but also what is likely to be seen as problematic about them.

At the same time a piece of research will entail a model of what people are like. At one extreme the form of conceptualization may embody a variety of **determinism**, treating people as the product of their inherent nature (biological determinism) or their immediate surroundings (environmental determinism, or behaviourism) or the history and structure of the social order (sociological determinism). At the other extreme, research may conceptualize people as free and autonomous agents (**voluntarism**) – the thinking, feeling, experiencing beings of some humanistic social psychology, or the imperfect, selfish and competing animals of some New Right conceptualizations. In between come notions of unconscious motivation, ideological influence, and a wide range of theories (interacting with the models of society outlined above) which look for interaction or articulation between the ways in which we may be conceived of as 'free' to decide and the ways in which we may be shown to be 'bound' and determined by factors extrinsic to our consciousness.

Models of the person are strongly reflected in the general styles into which research studies fall. Much quantitative, positivistic research assumes the person as in some way determined, a product of biology or upbringing or environment or social structure. It looks for the **causes** of events and behaviours, applying consistent stimuli in the assurance of eliciting consistent responses. Some qualitative work embodies a deterministic perspective, but it sees people as the product of their social environment – the people around them, the local consensus on norms and values, and/or wider social structures or ideologies. Some qualitative work, still deterministic, is framed in terms of 'inner forces' of which the conscious person may be unaware. Yet other kinds are framed in terms of actually or potentially autonomous people capable of understanding their lives and taking control of them. In all these varieties there is less interest in the supposed causes of behaviours, and more interest in the understanding and analysis of what aspects of the social or individual world mean for those who experience them.

A particular conflict of models – not a controversy, but something built into the basic way of looking at things – crops up when we try to do research which is in any sense collaborative and includes the 'subjects' or 'informants' as equal participants. Basic to the notion of collaborative research is a model of all people – not just the researcher – as knowledgeable about their own problems or at least prepared to explore what they may be in the same way as the researcher is prepared to explore them. In other words, the collaborative model assigns no particular expertise or knowledge to the researcher, over and above what he or she may happen to have read. The essence of the collaborative approach is that the researcher does not 'own' the research – that he or she is not, in fact, 'the researcher', but merely someone with particular skills or knowledge of literature who is prepared to share these skills. There is a further corollary: that this is how research should be, that any other way of approaching research is exploitative. This model is central to collaborative research of any kind; to the extent that the model does not describe what was going on, the research was not collaborative. On the other hand, there is an in-built tension: many who espouse this style also believe that we are not free to understand our situation except through education and 'consciousness raising'; people are deceived by the ideology inherent in their situation and need help to see beyond it. This tension between education and equal participation is entirely typical of collaborative research and is the source of many of its practical and ethical dilemmas.

The 'teaching' point we are trying to make from all this, however, is that *there is no possibility of escaping the effect of underlying models of society and of the person*. To the extent that we try to do 'value-free' research which has no political overtones and just looks to describe 'the facts', we impose common sense models of society and the person on our research. The disadvantage of the common sense approach – what 'stands to reason' or is seen as 'natural' – is that it is unanalysed. It may fairly represent what is going on. It may equally be prone to every ideological and habitual shortcut for avoiding disquieting analysis that the social setting may happen to offer at the time of the research. It is difficult enough to separate oneself from the presuppositions of 'management'. To separate oneself from one's own presuppositions is more difficult still, and yet it is an essential part of the 'research imagination'.

Most difficult of all is to separate oneself from the set of assumptions built into our everyday thought. We are not speaking here of **ideologies** – coherent attempts to present someone else's interests as one's own – but what Foucault and others have called **discourses**. A discourse is a way of speaking about things, a way of 'dividing up the ground'; however, the terms of the discourse are seldom value-neutral. What a discourse does is to 'capture the agenda', to declare what shall be taken for granted as important. When you feel that there is something wrong with a line of argument, but you find it difficult to put it into words, because the terms of the argument do not seem to lend themselves to your way of seeing things and you find yourself arguing 'against the self-evident', this is a sure sign that a conflict of discourses is taking place.

We might illustrate what we mean by discourse from the rhetoric surrounding any general election – the fight over whether taxation or economic success or defence capability or sensibility to the plight of the poor is to be seen as the mark of 'good government'. Another particularly good example may be built around the concept of family, and the life and life-rights of women. Women may be defined in any one of a set of discourse-laden terms.

1 *Women as wives* clearly have a 'duty to their husbands' – and the duty has sexual implications. The role of a 'wife' is to be an adjunct to her husband, which has strong implications for the place of women in the labour market.
2 *Women as mothers* clearly have a 'duty to their children' – and this duty may interfere with their sexual duty as wives. It is axiomatic that the welfare of children comes before all else, so that this way of viewing women also has strong implications for the place of women in the labour market.
3 *Women as adults* can be seen as having just the same rights and responsibilities as men as adults, including the right to work. However,
4 *Women as workers* have available to them a labour market which takes for granted that they will be constrained by their role as mothers and wives (nurturant, caring, willing and *inherently able* to take on a supportive role). It also takes for granted, largely, that they will be supported by some man and not in need of a 'family wage'. Thus the mostly female segment of the labour market is very different from the mostly male segment.

In other words, these are incompatible ways of framing the debates: what seems reasonable to say when talking about women as adults (equal citizens) somehow seems to make no sense when talking about women as mothers (people devoted to the care of children).

There is an inherent problem here in what is required of the good researcher. On the one hand, we are required to identify what is taken for granted in the way that problems are formulated for us (in the case of commissioned research) or by us (in the case of research which we ourselves initiate), and in the answers which our informants give us. It is our job to see behind the easy formulation of the problem to the questions that might have been asked, and behind the easy answer to questions to the answers that might have been given. At the same time, we are people of our own culture, class, gender, race, profession, etc., and it is unclear just how we are expected to see behind our preconceptions.

There is no simple or conclusive answer to this question, just as there is no simple or final way of doing the 'seeing behind'. There are two points which might give us hope, however.

1 There is no single 'discourse' – no single set of concepts which 'describe reality' – but a multiplicity of ways of framing the world. In the example above, for instance, we can conceptualize women as wives, as mothers and as adults, all different ways of structuring the social world with regard to gender, and the fact that there are these different ways allows us to some extent to stand back from all of them.
2 To the extent that we are 'determined' or 'caused' by the prevailing frames, this causal force may be 'quasi-causal' (Wellmer 1969; Sapsford and Thomas 1985) – determining only to the extent that we are not aware of it. The whole force of the idea of 'consciousness-raising' is that what seems natural and is normally taken for granted may be set aside (to some small extent at least) once we realize that there are other ways of formulating the problem. This kind of raising of consciousness is characteristic of the very best outcomes of the research process.

In conclusion

In conclusion, research is not some mysterious 'technical subject' to be mastered by years of study, but something which we all can do, something we all do already. Research is asking questions, looking to see what is going on, trying out what happens if we make this or that change. There *are* techniques, and it helps to know them, but they can all be mastered when they are needed – or you can obtain help from others who *do* know them (e.g. statisticians, computer experts) provided you know *about* them. The more research you do and read about, the more techniques you will know about and have in your 'toolbox' for planning the next project. The key to good research, however, does not lie in the techniques. Good research is the product of clear analysis of problems, clear specification of goals, careful design of fieldwork and thoughtful analysis and exposition afterwards. What lies between is just good, honest work.

At the same time, good research is something very difficult to achieve. It takes a very clear and logical mind, coupled with a great deal of imagination. You have to be able to see round your own taken-for-granted presuppositions, and those of other people, to find the most fruitful way to formulate the problem and the goals of the research. You have to think clearly about what could possibly be concluded from the data you intend to collect, what objections might be raised to these conclusions, and whether your procedures could be modified to increase the interpretability of the results and to overcome the likely objections. You need great insight into how people will react and a lively apprehension of what could harm them or cause them discomfort. You need the ability to put your own interpretation of the world aside and take on that of the informants, for the purpose of the research, while staying sufficiently marginal to it that it does not dominate your thinking entirely. Finally, you need to be able to put aside your preferred conclusions if the data do not bear them out. All of this is very difficult, and no one ever manages to achieve all of it. It is the goal, however, and most of us occasionally achieve some small part of it.

A final point is that research, as an attitude of mind, is not confined to methods classes and formal research projects. The attitude of mind which is needed for research is also needed for our day-to-day practice. The same principles which inform a major research project also inform our constant small-scale attempts to evaluate and improve our own practice.

Summary

1 The use of research techniques in the evaluation of policy and practice is not confined to formal 'evaluation studies'; the reflective practitioner uses them to monitor and improve performance.

2 Traditionally, evaluation studies have involved quantitative methods – experimental or **quasi-experimental** designs to test the effects of procedures, or surveys to gather opinions and intentions.

3 Open, qualitative methods are playing an increasing part in evaluation, however, and they are the only way to conduct research which can lay the basic paradigm of the research itself open to question.

4 No research is neutral, ethically and politically. Even if not 'applied' in the sense of aiming to develop or test a procedure, provision or policy, it is informed by (often unconscious) views about the nature of people and the social order and what these *should* be like. Unreflective research often serves to reproduce, maintain and justify the existing state of affairs.

5 Two good ethical principles to bear in mind when planning or assessing research are (a) that no one should be harmed or subjected to discomfort by the research, or even *feel* harmed or discommoded, and (b) that the full and informed consent of all participants should be obtained.

6 However, these 'rules' do not, in our view, solve all ethical dilemmas; often they function only as guidelines, and serious problems remain to be resolved.

7 Increasingly, researchers are questioning traditional modes of research and the assumption that the researcher has some kind of right to investigate problems, whatever the cost to those investigated and however intrusive the research. Increasingly researchers are emphasizing the political function of research and the researcher's ethical duty to take into account the interests of those who are researched. Many researchers argue that informed consent to the research should be obtained in all instances.

8 This sensitivity to the power relations inherent in research has led some people to argue that all research should be 'collaborative' – taking a problem of the researched and aimed at solving *that* problem in collaboration, or involving the collaboration of colleagues to carry out joint evaluation of their own practice – and not determined by a *researcher's*

interests. However, not all research which uses the rhetoric of collaboration is entirely collaborative in its design and purpose, nor does the collaborative paradigm suit every kind of researchable problem.

9 Where collaboration is not achievable, one might argue at least that the principle of informed consent ought to hold – that it is in keeping with the holistic nature of the professional stance in the caring professions. However, this does not absolve the researcher from responsibility, and from the need to exercise imagination and reflexive insight in the interests of or to protect the 'subjects' of research. The research relationship embodies an asymmetry of power (except in the almost unattainable ideal of fully collaborative research), and researchers have to consider the outcome of their work and the question of whose 'side' they are on.

Further reading

Shakespeare, Pamela, Atkinson, Dorothy and French, Sally (eds) (1993) *Reflecting on Research Practice: Issues in Health and Social Welfare*. Buckingham: Open University Press.

Smith, Dorothy (1987) *The Everyday World as Problematic*. Boston, MA: Northeastern Universities Press (Section 5, Researching the everyday world as problematic).

Bowles, Gloria and Klein, Renate (eds) (1983) *Theories of Women's Studies*. London: Routledge and Kegan Paul (articles by Klein, Du Bois, Mies, Reinharz, Stanley and Wise, Westcott, Evans).

Oja, Sharon and Smulyan, Lisa (1988) *Collaborative Action Research*. Basingstoke: Falmer.

Reason, Peter and Rowan, John (eds) (1981) *Human Inquiry: A Sourcebook of New Paradigm Research*. Chichester: Wiley.

Rose, Stephen and Black, Bruce (1985) *Advocacy and Empowerment*. London: Routledge and Kegan Paul.

Williams, Paul and Shoultz, Bonnie (1982) *We Can Speak for Ourselves*. London: Souvenir Press.

Abbott, Pamela and Wallace, Claire (1996) *An Introduction to Sociology: Feminist Perspectives*. London: Routledge.

Barrett, Michele (1988) *Women's Oppression Today* (2nd edition). London: Verso.

Billig, Michael *et al.* (1988) *Ideological Dilemmas: A Social Psychology of Everyday Thinking*. London: Sage.

Bryan, Beverley, Dadzie, Stella and Scafe, Fay (1985) *The Heart of the Race, Black Women's Lives in Britain*. London: Virago.

Commission for Racial Equality (1978) *Five Views of Multi-racial Britain*. London: CRE/BBC .

Pryce, Ken (1979) *Endless Pressure*. Harmondsworth: Penguin.

Shotter, John (1975) *Images of Man in Psychological Research*. London: Methuen.

GLOSSARY

Action research: evaluation of a practice or policy – often carried out by the practitioners – whose results are fed back into the policy or practice to modify it, leading to a further round of evaluation.

Alternative explanation: one which is equally as plausible, on the evidence presented, as the explanation which the researcher concludes is the correct one. See also **statistical control**.

Applied research: a term which has often been used to mean that a piece of research is intended to have immediate consequences for policy or practice – as opposed to *theoretical research*, which has immediate consequences only for academic theory. More recently the term *applied research* has been restricted to research which is intended to solve some particular problem and does not generalize beyond the immediate case; research which has application in more than the particular case is termed *strategic research*.

Association: see **correlation**.

Case control: see **quasi-experimental analysis**.

Causation: one variable (the *independent* or *explanatory* variable) is said to cause another (the *dependent* variable) when the two are **correlated**; the independent variable precedes the dependent one in time and a mechanism connecting the two can be demonstrated or is at least strongly suspected.

Census: a survey of a total population. *The* Census generally means the decennial census of the population of Great Britain and Northern Ireland.

Cluster sampling: sampling geographical units or clusters (e.g. whole classes within schools rather than a random sample of pupils irrespective of what class they are in), to cut down costs and/or travelling time. This can produce samples which are fairly representative of their populations – particularly if an element of randomness is introduced into the selection – but is likely to underestimate the variability of the population.

Cohort study: see **prospective study**.

Collaborative research: research in which the researcher and those being researched share the same aims and there is no differential of power or knowledge between the researcher and the researched.

Comparison group: a second group of research subjects as similar as possible to the first in every respect except one; it is used to try to eliminate alternative explanations.

Confidence limits: the range of values, estimated from the results for a single random sample, within which a given proportion of the values for repeated samples should lie (usually 95 per cent or 99 per cent).

Confounded variables: see **statistical control**.

Control group: see **comparison group**, **experiment**.

Controlled trial: see **experiment**.

Correlation: the common variation of two variables; variables are said to be *correlated* or *associated* when an individual's score on one variable predicts his or her score on another. *Positive correlation* is where high scores predict high scores – physical fitness predicting running speed, for example. *Negative correlation* is where high scores on one predict low scores on the other, and vice versa – physical fitness predicting likelihood of heart failure, for example. It is a truism of statistics that *correlation does not necessarily imply causation*.

Covert research: studies in which the fact that research is taking place (or, at least, its purpose) is concealed.

Critical analysis: analysis of text for underlying ideologies and models of the person and the social order, taking into account the circumstances of the text's production. See also **discourse analysis**.

Cross-sectional studies: studies which collect data at one point in time. Also known as **one-shot studies**.

Dependent variable: see **causation**.

Descriptive statistics: figures about a population (e.g. birth rates, death rates).

Design: the construction of a study, in terms of sampling and how data are collected, to minimize reactivity and ensure that variables are not confounded, in order to eliminate possible alternative explanations of the results. See also **experiment**, **reactivity**, **sampling**, **validity**.

Determinism: the belief that the whole of a person's behaviour can be accounted for by antecedent causes.

Discourse analysis: the analysis of text or speech, or indeed action patterns representable as text, in terms of ideologies (coherent groups of propositions which favour the interests of a dominant group but express themselves as in the interests of a subordinate group) and discourses (coherent patterns of 'rules' which specify the objects which may be discussed and the basis on which propositions made about them will be judged true or false).

Double-blind techniques: the administration of experimental treatments in such a way that neither the subject *nor the person administering the treatment* knows whether a given subject is in the experimental or the control group.

Epidemiology: the study of the origin and spread of medical or other conditions. See **quasi-experimental analysis**.

Expected values: in *inferential statistics*, the numbers that would be expected if distribution between categories was by chance alone and the supposed explanatory variables actually had no effect; in *descriptive statistics*, the numbers that would be expected if the group under study had the same composition as the population (for example, the expected deaths in a group during a time-period are calculated by taking account of the effect of age and gender on deaths in the population).

Experiment: research in which the researcher administers a measured treatment to one set of subjects, measuring a dependent variable before and after administration, and withholds the treatment from a similarly constituted *control group* (or constructs a control condition in some other way). Medical experiments in which a drug or other treatment is applied to a group of experimental subjects and withheld from a 'control group' are generally called *controlled trials*.

Field notes: in observation research, data recorded by the researcher during or immediately after each observation session, detailing what happened, what was said, probably how the researcher felt about it and possibly a preliminary attempt at analysis and any ideas which occurred to the researcher at the time of observing or writing the notes.

Haphazard sampling: see **opportunity sampling**.

Holism: the study of a natural or personal situation as a whole, rather than the sum of parts.

Ideology: see **discourse analysis**.

Independent variable: see **causation**.

Inferential statistics: techniques, based on the mathematics of probability, for (a) estimating population values from sample values, given random sampling, and (b) estimating the likelihood that a difference or correlation as large as the value obtained in a study could have arisen by chance sampling of a population in which the difference or correlation did not in fact exist. See also **sampling error**.

Interaction effect: a patterned variation observed sometimes when looking at the effects of more than one independent variable on a dependent variable, such that the effects are not additive but multiplicative – the effect of both independent variables together is larger than or, at least, different from what would be predicted from their separate effects.

Interview schedule: a list of questions to be administered by an interviewer.

Longitudinal studies: studies which collect data by repeated measurement over time. See also **time-series designs** and **panel studies**.

Market research: research carried out, generally by manufacturing/retail companies or specialist market research companies commissioned by them, to evaluate the market for a product or the effectiveness of an advertising campaign. The term is also used, more loosely, to include opinion surveys such as those carried out on behalf of major newspapers to assess the support in the country for a political party and its leader and policies.

Matched groups: (a) groups so selected as to have similar *average* values on variables known to affect the dependent variable, or (b) groups constituted by matching pairs of *individuals* on these variables and assigning them randomly to one group or the other. The latter process is more difficult to achieve but provides better evidence.

Natural experiment: see **quasi-experimental analysis**.

Naturalism: the principle of disturbing the 'natural situation' as little as possible.

New paradigm: a term coined by humanistic psychologists to refer to research which respects the individuality of those who are the 'subjects' of research; such studies are generally qualitative and collaborative in form.

Observation: research in which data are collected by recording what is seen/experienced. Observation may be *participant* (with the observer taking a role in the social setting and interacting with other participants) or *non-participant* (from behind a one-way window, for example, or by use of video equipment). Observation studies also differ in their degree of *structure*. Non-participant studies are generally highly structured, seeking to measure behaviour, while participant studies are generally relatively open, seeking to share experiences, but the connection between degree of structure and type of study is not invariant.

One-shot designs: see **cross-sectional studies**.

Open-ended questions: questions whose range of possible answers is not predetermined.

Operationalization: determining how a theoretical concept may validly be measured.

Opportunity sampling: using as sample a group which just happens to be available and accessible, without any thought as to whether it is representative of the population. Also known as *haphazard sampling*.

Overt research: research in which the existence of the research is acknowledged and its nature explained. See also **covert research**.

Panel studies: studies in which data are collected over time from a group of informants, the same informants being questioned or measured in each time period.

Pilot work: (generally small-scale) research undertaken to develop a measuring instrument, test the use of a questionnaire, try out experimental procedures, explore an observational setting or familiarize oneself with the language and concepts of a research population.

Prospective study: one which selects a group of people and 'follows them up' to see which factors measured early in the study predict variation in the dependent variable(s) under investigation; also known as *cohort studies*. The opposite is a *retrospective study*, where data are collected about the past of two groups now known to differ with respect to the dependent variable, with the intention of identifying explanatory variables.

Psychometrics: the measurement of personal characteristics and abilities, generally by means of 'paper and pencil' or performance tests.

Quasi-experimental analysis: the comparison of (often) 'naturally occurring' groups (e.g. smokers and non-smokers) as if they were experimental and control groups in a true experiment, looking for causal connections. In policy research this kind of comparison of groups which happen to have experienced or been excluded from the effects of a policy is sometimes called a *natural experiment*. In medical research the quasi-experimental comparison of cases with differing characteristics and outcomes is called *case control*. Lacking the control over allocation to groups given by the true experiment, this kind of analysis has to control for alternative explanations by statistical means. **Epidemiology** also works largely by quasi-experimental logic, isolating some variables as causal and eliminating others by means of statistical control. See **statistical control**.

Questionnaire: a list of questions to be answered by an informant. See also **interview schedule**.

Quota sampling: a non-random method of stratified sampling, where interviewers are sent to collect data from *quotas* of informants defined by variables likely to have an important effect on the dependent variable. The achieved sample will be representative of the population with respect to these variables but may not (indeed, is quite likely *not* to) be representative of the population in other respects.

Random: without discernible pattern or bias – selection by chance alone. *Random allocation*, in experiments, means allocation of subjects to experimental or control groups by random means. *Random sampling*, in surveys or other studies aiming to describe a population, means selecting the sample by chance alone (within the rules of the sampling design).

Reactivity: the elicitation of behaviour or speech by the research procedures – *personal reactivity* being differential reaction to the person and behaviour of the researcher, and *procedural reactivity* being variation in data caused by the structure of the study or the way questions are asked. Where a high degree of reactivity is present it is likely that observed differences between groups are due to the structure or conduct of the research, not to genuine underlying differences between the groups themselves.

Reductionism: the study of a personal or social situation by analysing its constituent parts.

Reflexivity: sensitivity to the research process itself, to possible reactivity and to the researcher's own biases. A *reflexive account* is an account of how the research was conducted, presented as an aid to assessing its validity.

Reliability: the consistency of a measuring instrument over time – an aspect of validity of measurement.

Replication: repeating a piece of research, on the grounds that a result is much less likely to have occurred by chance alone if it can be obtained more than once.

Representative: a sample is said to be representative of its population when the percentage distribution of traits in the sample predicts the distribution in the population, within calculable error limits. (See **confidence limits**.) A researched group which cannot be put forward as representative in this precise sense may nonetheless be typical of the population from which it is drawn – drawn from across the range rather than containing an untypically small number of kinds of case.

Retrospective study: see **prospective study**.

'Rhetoric': purposive speech, intended to produce an effect on the listener. In the narrow sense, 'rhetoric' is persuasive public speaking which aims to sell a political position to the audience, irrespective of whether the content of the speech is true or not. In a broader sense, it is what we say about public and political matters when we are describing how we think things ought to be or the consensus as to how they are; a 'rhetoric' bears no necessary relation to how the person employing it thinks, feels or acts.

Sampling: selecting a sub-group of a population from which to make inferences about the population as a whole. The best samples are drawn by **random**

methods, in order to ensure that every member of the population has a known, non-zero chance of being selected and that no bias on the part of the researcher is reflected in the composition of the sample.

Sampling error: an estimate of the likelihood that the true population value lies within a given distance of the value obtained from a random sample – the basis for calculating **confidence limits**, and also the basis of estimation in **inferential statistics**.

Secondary sources: data sources which were not compiled for the purpose of the research – government statistics, newspaper articles, departmental reports, diaries, letters, novels, etc.

SMR: see **standardized mortality ratio**.

Standardization: rendering figures comparable by calculating them on the same basis. The simplest case is percentaging.

Standardized mortality ratio: the deaths in a given area expressed as a ratio to the number that would be expected if the area had the same composition by age and gender as the national population and the same death rate. A figure of 100 means that the rates are the same; more than a hundred means that the area has more deaths than would be expected.

Statistical control: control of alternative explanations by statistical means rather than by the design of the experiment or survey. For example, if a treatment and a control group differ markedly in their gender composition, it might be necessary to analyse the results of the experiment separately for males and females, to show that any observed differences between the groups is not due to gender. Variables are said to be *confounded* when this kind of control is not possible; for example, we cannot separate, by statistical analysis, the effects of 'being biologically female' and 'having been socialized as a female'.

Strategic research: see **applied research**.

Stratification: in sampling, the process of dividing the population into bands or *strata* by one or more variables known to affect the dependent variable (typically social class, age, gender, ethnic group of origin) and sampling each group separately, in order to improve the precision of the population estimates.

Survey: a piece of research in which data are collected from a wide range of systematically sampled informants or subjects. Generally this involves asking questions of people, or administering tests, but the systematic collection of data from a sample of places or about a sample of objects would also be a survey.

Theoretical research: see **applied research**.

Theoretical sampling: the systematic study of further contexts or groups of individuals which differ from the first in known ways, to assess the generality of a model by seeing if they resemble or differ from the first in ways which the model would predict. See also **comparison group**.

Time-series designs: studies in which data are collected by repeated measurement over time, but different people are questioned or measured in the different time-periods.

Triangulation: using different sources of information to bear on and illuminate a single problem.

Trivialization: in quantitative research, the tendency for the important but vague to mutate, in the research design, into the less important but measurable.

Typicality: see **representative**.

Validity: (of a measurement technique) the degree to which the technique measures what it purports to measure; (of the design of a piece of research) the degree to which the conclusions of a study follow from the evidence it generates and the extent to which alternative explanations of the results have been or can be eliminated. See also **statistical control**.

Vignette: a description of a person, situation or event, used instead of 'the real thing' as a basis for discussion or judgement.

Voluntarism: the belief that not all of a person's behaviour can be accounted for by antecedent causes.

REFERENCES

Abbott, Pamela (1982) 'Towards a social theory of mental handicap', PhD thesis, Thames Polytechnic.

Abbott Pamela (1997) Home helps and district nurses: community care in the far South West, in P. Abbott and R. Sapsford (eds) *Research into Practice: A Reader for Nurses and the Caring Professions* (2nd edition). Buckingham: Open University Press.

Abbott, Pamela and Sapsford, Roger (1986) Diverse reports: caring for mentally handicapped children in the community, *Nursing Times*, 5 March: 47–9.

Abbott, Pamela and Sapsford, Roger (1987a) *Women and Social Class*. London: Tavistock.

Abbott, Pamela and Sapsford, Roger (1987b) *Community Care for Mentally Handicapped Children*. Milton Keynes: Open University Press. (Part is reprinted in Pamela Abbott and Roger Sapsford (1997) *Research into Practice: A Reader for Nurses and the Caring Professions* (2nd edition). Buckingham: Open University Press.)

Abbott, Pamela and Sapsford, Roger (1991) Health visiting: policing the family? in P. Abbott and C. Wallace (eds) *A Sociology of the Caring Professions*. Basingstoke: Falmer.

Abbott, Pamela and Sapsford, Roger (1993) Studying policy and practice: use of vignettes, *Nurse Researcher*, 1(2): 81–91. (Also reproduced in Pamela Abbott and Roger Sapsford (1997) *Research into Practice: A Reader for Nurses and the Caring Professions* (2nd edition). Buckingham: Open University Press.)

Abbott, Pamela and Sapsford, Roger (eds) (1997) *Research into Practice: A Reader for Nurses and the Caring Professions* (2nd edition). Buckingham: Open University Press.

Abbott, Pamela and Tyler, Melissa (1995) Ethnic variation in the female labour force: a research note, *British Journal of Sociology*, 46: 339–53. (Also reproduced in Pamela Abbott and Roger Sapsford (1997) *Research into Practice: A Reader for Nurses and the Caring Professions* (2nd edition). Buckingham: Open University Press.)

Abbott, Pamela and Wallace, Claire (1996) *An Introduction to Sociology: Feminist Perspectives* (2nd edition). London: Routledge.

Adelman, Clem and Alexander, Robin (1982) *The Self-evaluating Institution: Practice and Principles in the Management of Educational Change*. London: Methuen.

Anastasi, Anne (1982) *Psychological Testing*. London: Macmillan.

Arber, Sara and Ginn, Jay (1991) *Gender and Later Life: A Sociological Analysis of Resources and Constraints*. London: Sage.

Armitage, S. (1990) Research utilisation in practice, *Nurse Education Today*, 10(1): 10–15.

Backett, Kathryn (1982) *Mothers and Fathers*. London: Macmillan.

Bannister, Don and Fransella, Fay (1980) *Inquiring Man: The Theory of Personal Constructs*. Harmondsworth: Penguin.

Barrett, Michele (1988) *Women's Oppression Today: The Marxist/Feminist Encounter* (2nd edition). London: Verso.

Bayley, Michael (1973) *Mental Handicap and Community Care*. London: Routledge and Kegan Paul.

Billig, Michael *et al.* (1988) *Ideological Dilemmas: A Social Psychology of Everyday Thinking*. London: Sage.

Boon, J. (1995) From research to practice and back again. Paper presented at the

Royal College of Nursing Research Society Annual Conference at the University of Ulster.

Boulton, Mary (1983) *On Being a Mother*. London: Tavistock.

Bowles, Gloria and Klein, Renate (eds) (1983) *Theories of Women's Studies*. London: Routledge and Kegan Paul.

Breakwell, Glynnis, Foot, Hugh and Gilmour, Robin (eds) (1982) *Social Psychology: A Practical Manual*. London: Macmillan/British Psychological Society.

Briggs, A. (1972) *Report of the Committee on Nursing*. London: HMSO.

Brown, Dave and Kaplan, Robert (1981) Participative research in a factory, in P. Reason and J. Rowan (eds) *Human Inquiry: A Sourcebook of New Paradigm Research*. Chichester: Wiley.

Brown, George and Harris, Tirril (1978) *Social Origins of Depression: A Study of Psychiatric Disorder in Women*. London: Routledge and Kegan Paul.

Brown, Roswyn (1989) *Individualised Care: The Role of the Ward Sister*. Harrow: Scutari.

Bryan, Beverley, Dadzie, Stella and Scafe, Fay (1985) *The Heart of the Race: Black Women's Lives in Britain*. London: Virago.

Burgess, Robert (1984) *In the Field: An Introduction to Field Research*. London: Allen and Unwin.

Busfield, Joan (1991) *Women and Mental Health*. London: Macmillan.

Campbell, D.T. (1969) Reforms as experiments, *American Psychologist*, 24: 409–29.

Campbell, D.T. and Ross, H.L. (1968) The Connecticut crackdown: time-series data in quasi-experimental analysis, *Law and Society Review*, 3: 33–53.

Cartwright, A. (1979) *The Dignity of Labour?* London: Tavistock.

Caudill, W., Redlich, F.C., Gilmore, H. and Brody, E.B. (1952) Social structure and interaction processes on a psychiatric ward, *American Journal of Orthopsychiatry*, 22: 314–34.

Cavendish, Ruth (1982) *Women on the Line*. London: Routledge and Kegan Paul.

Cayne, Julia (1995) Portfolios: a developmental influence? in *Journal of Advanced Nursing*, 21: 395–405.

Central Statistical Office (periodically) *Guide to Official Statistics*. London: HMSO.

Clegg, Frances (1982) *Simple Statistics*. Cambridge: Cambridge University Press.

Commission for Racial Equality (1978) *Five Views of Multi-racial Britain*. London: CRE/BBC.

Cope, David (1981) *Organisational Development and Action Research in Hospitals*. Aldershot: Gower.

Cornwell, Jocelyn (1984) *Hard-Earned Lives: Accounts of Health and Illness from East London*. London: Tavistock.

Davies, Bleddyn, Bebbington, A. and Charnely, Helen (1990) *Resources, Needs and Outcomes in Community-Based Care*. Aldershot: Gower.

Davis, Fred (1963) *Passage through Crisis: Polio Victims and their Families*. Indianapolis, IN: Bobbs-Merril.

Department of Health (1991) *Research for Health: A Research Development Strategy for the National Health Service*. London: HMSO.

Dingwall, Robert and Fox, Susan (1986) Health visitors' and social workers' perceptions of child care problems, in A. While (ed.) *Research in Preventive Community Nursing Care: Fifteen Studies in Health Visiting*. Chichester: Wiley.

Dixon, Penelope (1967) 'Reduced emotional responsiveness in schizophrenia', PhD thesis, University of London.

Doll, Richard and Hill, A. Bradford (1950) Smoking and carcinoma of the lung: a preliminary report, *British Medical Journal*, 4682: 739–48.

Doll, Richard and Hill, A. Bradford (1954) The mortality of doctors in relation to their smoking habits: a preliminary report, *British Medical Journal*, 4877: 1451–5.

Doll, Richard and Hill, A. Bradford (1956) Lung cancer and other causes of death in relation to smoking: a second report on the mortality of British doctors, *British Medical Journal*, 5001: 1071–81.

Doll, Richard and Hill, A. Bradford (1964) Mortality in relation to smoking: ten years' observation of British doctors, *British Medical Journal*, 5395: 1399–410 and 1460–7.

Doll, Richard and Peto, Richard (1981) *The Causes of Cancer: Quantitative Estimates of Avoidable Risks of Cancer*. Oxford: Oxford University Press.

Dominelli, Lena and McLeod, Eileen (1989) *Feminist Social Work*. London: Macmillan.

Drennan, Vari (1986) Talking to health visitors – perceptions of their work, in A. While (ed.) *Research in Preventive Community Nursing Care*. Chichester: Wiley.

Elden, Max (1979) Bank employees begin to participate in studying and changing their organisation, in International Organisation for the Quality of Working Life, *Working on the Quality of Working Life*. The Hague: Martinus Nijhoff.

Elden, Max (1981) Sharing the research work: participative research and its role demands, in P. Reason and J. Rowan (eds) *Human Inquiry: A Sourcebook of New Paradigm Research*. Chichester: Wiley.

Foucault, Michel (1963) *The Birth of the Clinic*. London: Tavistock 1973.

Foucault, Michel (1975) *Discipline and Punish: The Birth of the Prison*. London: Allen Lane 1977.

Foucault, Michel (1976) *The History of Sexuality, vol. I*. London: Allen Lane 1979.

Fransella, Fay and Frost, K. (1977) *On Being a Woman*. London: Tavistock.

Fulani, Lenora (ed.) (1988) *The Politics of Race and Gender in Therapy*. New York: Haworth Press.

Garrett, G. (1990) *Older People: Their Support and Care*. Basingstoke: Macmillan.

Giovannoni, J.M. and Becerra, R.M. (1979) *Defining Child Abuse*. London: Collier Macmillan.

Glaser, Barry and Strauss, Anselm (1967) *The Discovery of Grounded Theory*. Chicago, IL: Aldine.

Glendinning, Carolyn (1983) *Unshared Care: Parents and their Disabled Children*. London: Routledge and Kegan Paul.

Goffman, Erving (1961) *Asylums: Essays on the Social Situation of Mental Patients and Other Inmates*. New York: Anchor Books (also Harmondsworth: Penguin).

Goffman, Erving (1963) *Stigma: The Management of Spoilt Identities*. New York: Anchor Books (also Harmondsworth: Penguin).

Goldthorpe, J.H., Lockwood, D., Bechhofer, F. and Platt, J. (1969) *The Affluent Worker in the Class Structure*. Oxford: Oxford University Press.

Gordon, Verona (1982) Themes and cohesiveness observed in depressed women's support group, *Issues in Mental Health Nursing*, 4: 115–25.

Gordon, Verona (1986) Treatment of depressed women by nurses in Britain and the USA, in J. Brooking (ed.) *Psychiatric Nursing Research*. Chichester: Wiley.

Gordon, Verona and Ledray, L. (1984) The alleviation of subclinical depression in women of middle years (unpublished).

Hakim, Catherine (1987) *Research Design: Strategies and Choices in the Design of Social Research*. London: Routledge.

Hammersley, Martyn and Atkinson, Paul (1995) *Ethnography: Principles in Practice* (2nd edition). London: Routledge.

Hammick, Marilyn (1996) *Managing the Ethical Process in Research*. Salisbury: Quay Books.

Haskey, John (1989) Families and households of the ethnic minority and white populations of Great Britain, *Population Trends*, 57: 8–19.

Heron, John (1973) *Re-evaluation Counselling: A Theoretical Review*. Guildford: University of Surrey Human Potential Research Project.

Heron, John (1977) *Behaviour Analysis in Education and Training*. Guildford: University of Surrey Human Potential Research Project.

Heron, John (1978) *An ASC Peer Research Group*. Guildford: University of Surrey Human Potential Research Project.

Heron, John (1979) *Peer Review Audit*. Guildford: University of Surrey Human Potential Research Project.

Heron, John (1981) Self and peer assessment for managers, in T. Boydell and M. Pedler (eds) *Handbook of Management Self Development*. London: Gower.

Hersen, Michael and Barlow, David (1976) *Single-Case Experimental Designs: Strategies for Studying Behavioural Change*. Oxford: Pergamon.

Hindess, Barry (1973) *The Use of Official Statistics in Sociology*. London: Macmillan.

Hollander, Edwin (1981) *Principles and Methods of Social Psychology*. Oxford: Oxford University Press.

Hollway, Wendy (1989) *Subjectivity and Method in Psychology: Gender, Meaning and Science*. London: Sage.

Hollway, Wendy (1991) *Work Psychology and Organisational Behaviour: Managing the Individual*. London: Sage.

Home Office (annual) *Statistics of Death Reported to Coroners*. London: HMSO.

Horsley, J.A., Crane, J., Crabtree, M.K. and Wood, A.J. (1983) *Using Research to Improve Nursing Practice: A Guide*. New York: Grune and Stratton.

Hunt, J.M. (1981) Indicators for nursing practice: the use of research findings, *Journal of Advanced Nursing*, 6: 189–94.

Hunt, J.M. (1996) Guest editorial, *Journal of Advanced Nursing*, 23: 423–5.

Hyener, R.H. (1985) Some guidelines for the phenomenological analysis of interview data, *Human Problems*, 8: 279–303.

Irvine, John, Miles, Ian and Evans, Jeff (eds) (1979) *Demystifying Social Statistics*. London: Pluto Press.

Jackins, H. (1965) *The Human Side of Human Beings: The Theory of Re-evaluation Counselling*. Seattle: Rational Island Publishers.

James, Nicky (1984) A postscript to nursing, in C. Bell and H. Roberts (eds) *Sociological Research: Politics, Problems, Practice*. London: Routledge and Kegan Paul. (A slightly shortened version is reprinted in Abbott and Sapsford (1997) *Research into Practice: A Reader for Nurses and the Caring Professions* (2nd edition). Buckingham: Open University Press.)

Jamieson, A. (ed.) (1991) *Home Care for Older People in Europe*. Oxford: Oxford University Press.

Jefferys, M. (ed.) (1989) *Growing Old in the Twentieth Century*. London: Routledge.

Jensen, Arthur (1981) *Straight Talk about Mental Tests*. London: Macmillan.

Kamin, Leon (1974) *The Science and Politics of I.Q.* New York: Erlbaum (also Harmondsworth: Penguin 1977).

Kazdin, Alan (1982) *Single-Case Research Design: Methods for Clinical and Applied Settings*. Oxford: Oxford University Press.

Kelly, George (1955) *The Psychology of Personal Constructs*. New York: Norton.

Kemmis, S. and McTaggart, R. (1982) *The Action Research Planner*. Deakin: University of Deakin Press.

Kenner, Charmian (1985) *No Time for Women: Exploring Women's Health in the 1930s and Today*. London: Pandora.

Kirkham, Mavis (1983) Labouring in the dark: limitations on the giving of information to enable patients to orient themselves to the likely events and timescale of labour, in J. Wilson-Barnett (ed.) *Nursing Research: Ten Studies in Patient Care*. Chichester: Wiley. (A slightly shortened version is reprinted in Abbott and Sapsford (1997) *Research into Practice: A Reader for Nurses and the Caring Professions* (2nd edition). Buckingham: Open University Press.)

Kitzinger, Sheila (1978) *Women as Mothers*. London: Fontana.

Knight, Barry and West, Donald (1975) Temporary and continuing delinquency, *British Journal of Criminology*, 15: 43.

Kratz, Charlotte (ed.) (1979) *The Nursing Process*. London: Bailliere Tindall.

Lorenson, Margarethe (1983) Effects of touch in patients during a crisis situation in hospital, in J. Wilson-Barnett (ed.), *Nursing Research: Ten Studies in Patient Care*. Chichester: Wiley.

Lucker, J. (1992) Research and development in nursing, *Journal of Advanced Nursing*, 17(10): 1151–2.

McClelland, D., Atkinson, V.W., Clarke, R.A. and Lowell, E.L. (1953) *The Achievement Motive*. New York: Appleton Century.

McCracken, Grant (1988) *The Long Interview*. Beverly Hills, CA: Sage.

McKee, Paul (1981) Statistics of politics, in Open University Course D291, *Statistical Sources*. Milton Keynes: The Open University.

McLeod, C.J. and Slodatski, A.N. (1978) How to find out: a guide to searching the nursing literature, *Nursing Times*, 74(6): 21–3.

McNiff, J. (1988) *Action Research: Principles and Practice*. London: Macmillan.

Marsh, Catherine (1982) *The Survey Method: The Contribution of Surveys to Sociological Explanation*. London: Allen and Unwin.

Marsh, Catherine (1988) *Exploring Data: An Introduction to Data Analysis for Social Scientists*. Cambridge: Polity.

Maternity Services Advisory Committee (1984) *Maternity Care in Action Pt II: Care during Childbirth*. London: HMSO.

Maternity Services Advisory Committee (1985) *Maternity Care in Action Pt III: Care of the Mother and Baby*. London: HMSO.

Metcalf, Clare (1983) A study of change in the method of organising the delivery of nursing care in a ward of a maternity hospital, in J. Wilson-Barnett (ed.) *Nursing Research: Ten Studies in Patient Care*. Chichester: Wiley.

Mies, Maria (1983) Towards a methodology for feminist research, in G. Bowles and R. Klein (eds) *Theories of Women's Studies*. London: Routledge and Kegan Paul.

Mitchell, J. Clyde (1983) Case and situation analysis, *Sociological Review*, 31: 187–211.

Nairn, Kathy and Smith, Gerrilyn (1984) *Dealing with Depression*. London: Women's Press.

Newmark, Charles (1985) *Major Psychological Assessment Instruments*. Boston, MA: Allyn and Bacon.

Oakley, Ann (1972) *Sex, Gender and Society*. London: Fontana.

Oakley, Ann (1980) *Women Confined: Towards a Sociology of Childbirth*. Oxford: Martin Robertson.

Oakley, Ann (1981) *From Here to Maternity*. Harmondsworth: Penguin.

Office of Population Censuses and Surveys (various) *OPCS Monitor*. London: OPCS.

Office of Population Censuses and Surveys (annual) *Population Trends*. London: HMSO.

Office of Population Censuses and Surveys (annual) *Social Trends*. London: HMSO.

Oja, Sharon and Smulyan, Lisa (1988) *Collaborative Action Research: A Developmental Process*. Basingstoke: Falmer.

Oppenheim, A.N. (1992) *Questionnaire Design, Interviewing and Attitude Measurement*. London: Pinter.

Orr, Jean (1986) Working with women's health groups: the community health movement, in A. While (ed.) *Research in Preventive Community Nursing: Fifteen Studies in Health Visiting*. Chichester: Wiley.

Osgood, Charles, Sui, George and Tannenbaum, Percy (1967) *The Measurement of Meaning*. Urbana, IL: University of Illinois Press.

Patton, Michael (1987) *How to Use Qualitative Methods in Evaluation*. Beverly Hills, CA: Sage.

Pearcey, P. (1995) Achieving research-based nursing practice, *Journal of Advanced Nursing*, 22: 33–9.

Penfold, Susan and Walker, Gillian (1984) *Women and the Psychiatric Paradox*. Milton Keynes: Open University Press.

Phillipson, C., Bernard, M. and Strang, P. (eds) (1986) *Dependency and Interdependency in Old Age: Theoretical Perspectives and Policy Alternatives*. Beckenham: Croom Helm.

Plummer, Kenneth (1983) *Documents of Life: An Introduction to the Problems and Literature of a Humanistic Method*. London: Allen and Unwin.

Polgar, Stephen and Thomas, Shane (1988) *Introduction to Research in the Health Sciences*. London: Churchill Livingstone.

Porter, Marilyn (1983) *Home, Work and Class Consciousness*. Manchester: Manchester University Press.

Potter, Jonathan and Wetherell, Margaret (1987) *Discourse and Social Psychology: Beyond Attitudes and Behaviour*. London: Sage.

Pryce, Ken (1979) *Endless Pressure: A Study of West Indian Life-styles in Bristol*. Harmondsworth: Penguin.

Reason, Peter (1981) An exploration of the dialectics of two-person relationships, in P. Reason and J. Rowan (eds) *Human Inquiry: A Sourcebook of New Paradigm Research*. Chichester: Wiley.

Reason, Peter and Rowan, John (eds) (1981) *Human Inquiry: A Sourcebook of New Paradigm Research*. Chichester: Wiley.

Reinharz, Shulamit (1979) *On Becoming a Social Scientist*. San Francisco, CA: Jossey-Bass.

Reinharz, Shulamit (1983) Experiential analysis: a contribution to feminist research, in G. Bowles and R. Klein (eds) *Theories of Women's Studies*. London: Routledge and Kegan Paul.

Roethlisberger, F.J. and Dickson, W.J. (1939) *Management and the Worker*. Cambridge, MA: Harvard University Press.

Rogers, A. (1992) *Adults Learning for Development*. London: Cassell.

Rose, Nikolas (1985) *The Psychological Complex*. London: Routledge and Kegan Paul.

Rose, Nikolas (1989) *Governing the Soul: The Shaping of the Private Self*. London: Routledge.

Rose, Stephen and Black, Bruce (1985) *Advocacy and Empowerment: Mental Health Care in the Community*. London: Routledge and Kegan Paul.

Ross, H.L. and Campbell, D.T. (1968) The Connecticut speed crackdown: a study of the effects of legal change, in H.L. Ross (ed.) *Perspectives on the Social Order: Readings in Sociology*. New York: McGraw-Hill.

Roth, Julius (1963) *Timetables*. Indianapolis, IN: Bobbs-Merril.

Sapsford, Roger (1983) *Life-sentence Prisoners: Reaction, Response and Change*. Milton Keynes: Open University Press.

Sapsford, Roger and Thomas, Kerry (1985) Change the individual and the social world, in Block 7 of Open University course D307, *Social Psychology: Development, Experience and Behaviour*. Milton Keynes: The Open University.

Savage, Wendy (1986) *A Savage Enquiry: Who Controls Childbirth?* London: Virago.

Schön, D. (1987) *Educating the Reflective Practitioner*. San Francisco, CA: Jossey-Bass.

Shakespeare, Pamela, Atkinson, Dorothy and French, Sally (eds) (1993) *Reflecting on Research Practice: Issues in Health and Social Welfare*. Buckingham: Open University Press.

Shearer, Anne (1972) *A Report on Public and Professional Attitudes towards the Sexual and Emotional Attitudes of Handicapped People*. London: Spastics Society/National Association for Mental Handicap.

Sherlock, Effie (1987) The Liverpool experience: the Croxteth Women's Health Group – self-help on a deprived community of Liverpool, in Jean Orr (ed.) *Women's Health in the Community*. Chichester: Wiley.

Shotter, John (1975) *Images of Man in Psychological Research*. London: Methuen.

Smith, Dorothy (1987) *The Everyday World as Problematic: A Feminist Sociology*. Boston, MA: Northeastern Universities Press.

Smith, Jonathan, Harre, Rom and Van Langenhove, Luk (1995) *Rethinking Methods in Social Psychology*. London: Sage.

Tandon, Rajesh (1981) Dialogue as enquiry and intervention, in P. Reason and J. Rowan (eds) *Human Inquiry: A Sourcebook of New Paradigm Research*. Chichester: Wiley.

Taylor, S.J. and Bogden R. (1984) *An Introduction to Qualitative Research Methods: The Search for Meanings*. Chichester: Wiley.

Torbert, William (1981) A collaborative enquiry into voluntary metropolitan desegregation, in P. Reason and J. Rowan (eds) *Human Inquiry: A Sourcebook of New Paradigm Research*. Chichester: Wiley.

Voysey, M. (1975) *A Constant Burden: The Reconstitution of Family Life*. London: Routledge and Kegan Paul.

Walsh, M. and Ford, P. (1989) *Nursing Rituals*. Oxford: Heinemann.

Wasoff, F. (1992) Simulated clients in 'natural' settings: constructing a client to study professional practice, *Sociology*, 26: 333–49.

Waterman, H., Webb, C. and Williams, A. (1995) Parallels and contradictions in the theory and practice of action research and nursing, *Journal of Advanced Nursing*, 22: 779–84.

Webb, C. (1992) The use of the first person in academic writing: objectivity, language and gatekeeping, *Journal of Advanced Nursing*, 17: 747–52.

Wellmer, Albrecht (1969) *Critical Theory of Society*. New York: Herder and Herder.

West, D.J. (1969) *Present Conduct and Future Delinquency*. London: Heinemann.

West, D.J. (1973) *Who Becomes Delinquent?* London: Heinemann.

Wetherell, Margaret (1995) Romantic discourse: analysing power, investment and desire, in S. Wilkinson and C. Kitzinger (eds) *Feminism and Discourse*. London: Sage.

Wetherell, Margaret and Potter, Jonathan (1992) *Mapping the Language of Racism: Discourse and the Legitimation of Exploitation*. Hemel Hempstead: Harvester/Wheatsheaf.

Williams, Anne (1987) Making sense of feminist contributions to women's health, in Jean Orr (ed.) *Women's Health in the Community*. Chichester: Wiley.

Williams, Paul and Shoultz, Bonnie (1982) *We Can Speak for Ourselves: Self Advocacy by Mentally Handicapped People*. London: Souvenir Press.

Wilson-Barnett, Jenifer and Robinson, Sarah (eds) (1989) *Directions in Nursing Research*. Harrow: Scutari.

Witts, L.J. (ed.) (1964) *Medical Surveys and Clinical Trials*. London: Oxford University Press.

AUTHOR INDEX

SUBJECT INDEX

RESEARCH INTO PRACTICE (SECOND EDITION)
A READER FOR NURSES AND THE CARING PROFESSIONS

Pamela Abbott and Roger Sapsford (eds)

Praise for the first edition of *Research into Practice and Research Methods for Nurses and the Caring Professions*:

> These books provide a good introduction for the uninitiated to reading and doing research. Abbott and Sapsford provide a clearly written and accessible introduction to social research . . . One of their aims is to 'de-mystify' research, and in this they succeed admirably . . . After reading the text and the articles in the reader, and working through the various research exercises, readers should have a clear appreciation of how to evaluate other people's research and how to begin their own.
>
> David Field, *Journal of Palliative Medicine*

This is a thoroughly revised and updated edition of the bestselling Reader for nurses and the caring professions. It offers carefully selected examples of research, all concerned in some way with nursing or the study of health and community care. It illustrates the kind of research that can be done by a small team or a single researcher, without large-scale research grants. The editors have chosen papers which show a great diversity of approaches: differing in emphasis on description or explanation, different degrees of structure in design and different appeals to the authority of science or the authenticity of emphatic exploration. They show the limitations typical of small-scale projects carried out with limited resources and the experience of applied research as it occurs in practice, as opposed to how it tends to look when discussed in textbooks. The chapters have been organized into three sections representing three distinct types of social science research: observing and participating, talking to people and asking questions, and controlled trials and comparisons. Each section is provided with an editorial introduction.

Contents
Introduction – Section A: Observing and participating – Labouring in the dark: limitations on the giving of information to enable patients to orient themselves to the likely events and timescale of labour – Portfolios: a developmental influence? – A postscript to nursing – Section B: Talking to people and asking questions – Leaving it to mum: community care for mentally handicapped children – Planning research: a case of heart disease – Home helps and district nurses: community care in the far South-west – Studying policy and practice: use of vignettes – Section C: Controlled trials and comparisons – Treatment of depressed women by nurses in Britain – The mortality of doctors in relation to their smoking habits: a preliminary report – Ethnic variation in the female labour force: a research note – Postscript – Author index – Subject index.

The Contributors
Pamela Abbott, Julia V. Cayne, Richard Doll, Verona Gordon, A. Bradford Hill, Nicky James, Mavis Kirkham, Roger Sapsford, Melissa Tyler.

184pp   0 335 19695 0 (Paperback)   0 335 19696 9 (Hardback)

PSYCHOLOGY FOR NURSES AND THE CARING PROFESSIONS

Sheila Payne and Jan Walker

- What is psychology and how is it relevant to health care practice?
- What influence do psychological factors have in determining outcomes in health care?
- What are the different approaches within psychology which can be used to understand normal human functioning?

Psychology for Nurses and the Caring Professions is one of a series of texts which provide coherent and multi-disciplinary support for all professional groups involved in the provision of health and social care. It introduces students to a range of psychological theories and research, supported by evidence from health psychology. Applications are offered within a variety of health care settings, with an emphasis on health promotion and preventive care.

The authors draw upon their clinical, teaching and research experience to engage the student's interest through the use of case examples, special research-based topics and exercises for group discussion or individual study. The text has been carefully designed with the student in mind: a comprehensive reference list is provided at the end of the book, together with a glossary of terms. The text is illustrated throughout with diagrams, tables and graphs, and suggestions for further reading are given at the end of each chapter.

Psychology for Nurses and the Caring Professions is a key textbook for all students undertaking diploma or degree level courses in nursing, health and social care.

Contents
Introduction to psychology – Understanding health and illness – Self concept and body image – Theories of learning: developments and applications – Perception, memory and patient information-giving – Stress and coping: theory and applications in health care – Development and loss in social relationships – Pain – Social processes in health care delivery – Epilogue – Glossary – References – Index.

240pp   0 335 19410 9 (Paperback)   0 335 19411 7 (Hardback)

SOCIAL POLICY FOR NURSES AND THE CARING PROFESSIONS

Louise Ackers and Pamela Abbott

- What is the relationship between social policy and health?
- Who provides social welfare?
- How has the provision of welfare developed?

Social Policy for Nurses and the Caring Professions is one of a series of texts which provide coherent and multi-disciplinary support for all professional groups involved in the provision of health and social care. It provides the student with a lively, readable and well illustrated introduction to social policy. The authors take as a starting point the importance of the conceptual connection between health and illness. The stress throughout the book is on the significance of social policy in preventing ill health and disability as well as supporting the sick and disabled. A broad approach to social policy is taken, and the text is organized around the provision of welfare in the following contexts:

- public
- private
- voluntary
- informal

Consideration is given to competing ideologies of welfare and the development of welfare as well as contemporary provision.

Social Policy for Nurses and the Caring Professions is based on the authors' first-hand teaching and research experience. The text has been carefully designed with the student in mind: a comprehensive reference list is provided at the end of the book, together with a glossary of important terms. The text is illustrated with tables and graphs throughout, and there are suggestions for further reading at the end of each chapter.

Social Policy for Nurses and the Caring Professions is a key textbook for all students undertaking diploma or degree level courses in nursing, health and social care.

Contents
What is social policy? – The development of a welfare state – Health inequalities and state health policies – Poverty, inequality and social policy – State income maintenance and welfare benefits – Privatization and social welfare – The changing role of the voluntary sector in the provision of social welfare – The role of informal care – The mixed economy of care: welfare services for dependent people – Welfare pluralism in the 1990s: the changing role of the state – Glossary – References – Index.

288pp   0 335 19359 5 (Paperback)   0 335 19360 9 (Hardback)